Health Promotion Ethics

Health Promotion Ethics: A Framework for Social Justice critically considers the ethical dimensions of promoting health with individuals and communities, encouraging a nuanced understanding of health promotion in the context of fairness, empowerment and social justice.

The concept of social justice, indeed, is central. The book explores how health promotion should be considered in relation to moral, social and legal issues, from individual responsibility to government intervention, as well as the possibility that existing practice maintains rather than alleviates existing health inequalities by stigmatising certain groups. It also questions the 'rights' of those who promote health to use particular strategies, for example using fear to encourage behaviour change. The ethics of health promotion practice and research are considered, introducing several important debates.

Case studies, international material and opportunities to reflect on practice are used throughout to bring the important issues under discussion to life, engaging both students and practitioners alike. The book provides a fascinating route to reflect on what it really means to promote health for all in a more equitable way.

Ruth Cross is Course Director in Health Promotion at Leeds Beckett University. Her research interests include qualitative and creative methods of investigation, feminist and critical perspectives, and the relationship between theory and practice. Ruth has edited and co-authored several textbooks, including *The Essentials of Health Promotion* (2022), *Health Promotion: Global Principles and Practice* (2021), *Health Promotion: Planning and Strategies* (2019) and *Health Communication: Theoretical and Critical Perspectives* (2017).

Louise Warwick-Booth is Reader and Associate Director of the Centre for Health Promotion Research. She leads a range of diverse research and evaluation projects with the voluntary and statutory sector. Her expertise relates to the evaluation of health promotion interventions with vulnerable populations, including women experiencing domestic abuse. Louise has published several textbooks such as *Social Inequality* (2022), *Creating Participatory Research* (2021) and *Contemporary Health Studies: An Introduction* (2021).

James Woodall is Reader in Health Promotion and Departmental Lead at Leeds Beckett University. James' research interest is the health-promoting prison and how values central to health promotion are applied to the context of imprisonment. He is currently Editor-in-Chief of the journal *Health Education*. James has published several textbooks such as *The Essentials of Health Promotion* (2022), *Practical Health Promotion* (2020) and *Health Promotion: Planning and Strategies* (2019).

Health Promotion Ethics
A Framework for Social Justice

Ruth Cross, Louise Warwick-Booth
and James Woodall

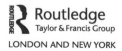

Routledge
Taylor & Francis Group

LONDON AND NEW YORK

Designed cover image: © Getty Images

First published 2024
by Routledge
4 Park Square, Milton Park, Abingdon, Oxon OX14 4RN

and by Routledge
605 Third Avenue, New York, NY 10158

Routledge is an imprint of the Taylor & Francis Group, an informa business

British Library Cataloguing-in-Publication Data
A catalogue record for this book is available from the British Library

Library of Congress Cataloging-in-Publication Data
Names: Cross, Ruth, author. | Warwick-Booth, Louise, author. | Woodall, James, author.
Title: Health promotion ethics : a framework for social justice / Ruth Cross, Louise Warwick-Booth, James Woodall.
Description: Abingdon, Oxon ; New York, NY : Routledge, 2024. | Includes bibliographical references and index.
Identifiers: LCCN 2023022138 | ISBN 9781032311500 (hardback) | ISBN 9781032311432 (paperback) | ISBN 9781003308317 (ebook)
Subjects: LCSH: Health promotion--Moral and ethical aspects. | Social justice--Health aspects.
Classification: LCC RA427.8 .C765 2024 | DDC 362.1--dc23/eng/20230710
LC record available at https://lccn.loc.gov/2023022138

ISBN: 978-1-032-31150-0 (hbk)
ISBN: 978-1-032-31143-2 (pbk)
ISBN: 978-1-003-30831-7 (ebk)

DOI: 10.4324/9781003308317

Typeset in Sabon LT Pro
by KnowledgeWorks Global Ltd.

Contents

Tables

Case studies

Preface

This book came about because we, the authors, perceived a gap in the literature around the health promotion ethics. Whilst there are some books around that consider the ethics of public health and, indeed, some book chapters with health promotion texts that focus on health promotion ethics, there did not seem to be anything that explored ethics in relation to health promotion in more depth. *Health Promotion Ethics: A Framework for Social Justice* positions health promotion as related to, but distinct from, public health. Given this distinct identity, we believe that a specific exploration of ethics and the application of ethical principles is warranted. The primary purpose of this book is to explore ethics in health promotion in relation to several different areas including practice, research and evaluation. We tackle many sticky issues that occur in the promotion of health such as debates about who is responsible for health, the wider, social determinants of health, and questions around whether the ends justify the means when we are seeking better health for all.

Drawing on our own research and practice in health promotion, the teaching and learning we facilitate on the suite of health promotion courses that we deliver at Leeds Beckett University, and on international literature we bring to life some of the ethical dilemmas faced in the promotion of health, including critiques of targeted interventions. Each chapter provides real-life *Case Studies* through which the reader can better appreciate some of the issues under discussion. *Reflection on Practice* opportunities are also dotted through the book which give readers a chance to pause, reflect and think about how the issues and debates might apply to their own practice.

It is hoped that *Health Promotion Ethics: A Framework for Social Justice* will encourage the reader to think about how they might promote health in a fairer and more ethical way. We will grapple with key questions throughout the text. Questions such as 'At what point should the state (government) intervene to protect individual health?', 'Who is responsible for health?', 'To what extent do well-meaning health promotion interventions stigmatise and marginalise people, or even worse, increase health inequalities?', 'Is it right to adopt fear strategies in health communication approaches?', 'Are the approaches we use always proportionate and useful?' and 'How do we carry out ethical research in health promotion?'.

Chapter 1 provides an overview of health promotion and is designed to give those who are relatively new to health promotion a good sense of what it is about to set the context for the rest of the book. The chapter should also serve as a useful reminder to those who already have some understanding of health promotion. It details our perspective in health promotion, setting out how we see health promotion as distinct from, although part of, broader public health. The discussion centres on three core values in health promotion – social justice, equity and empowerment. The issue of social justice is explored in relation to the social determinants of health as a platform for considering ethics in more detail in subsequent chapters. Key principles of health promotion are introduced in this chapter. Finally, individual and structural approaches to health promotion are considered. There are two case studies in this chapter – one about health inequalities in the United States and the other about road traffic injury, a global health issue.

Chapter 2 considers ethics as a key concern for health promotion generally as well as discussing some of the issues that health promotion faces from a philosophical perspective. It begins by considering what we understand by ethics moving onto a discussion about why ethics is a key component of health promotion, and why it is important to consider ethics in relation to health promotion. The chapter returns to the values and principles outlined in the previous one and explores the central role that ethics play in promoting health, outlining why ethics is positioned as a primary feeder discipline for health promotion by Bunton and Macdonald (2004). Several ethical frameworks are presented and discussed, such as Beauchamp and Childress' (2019) biomedical ethical principles. The chapter highlights how a biomedical understanding of ethics cannot easily be applied to health promotion's social model of health given biomedicine's attendant focus on individual responsibility and behaviour change. Sindall's (2002) notion of communitarian ethics is presented which takes into account common good, not simply the rights of the individual. The chapter ends with a longer case study on COVID-19.

Chapter 3 explores some of the key ethical debates in health promotion. Issues such as rights and responsibilities, structure and agency, the role of the state in the promotion of health, and the potential limits of autonomy are discussed. Using the Nuffield Ladder of Intervention as a framework, the chapter considers questions such as 'When is it right to intervene?', 'Is there a limit to personal choice?' and 'Does the greater good override the right to personal freedom?'. The chapter will outline and look at a number of tensions in these debates and there will be an in-depth exploration of Nudge Theory and Choice Architecture both of which have more recently been used in behaviour science as a means of promoting health and both of which raise several ethical issues worth exploring. Gregg and O'Hara's (2007) values and principles in the ethical and technical domains are also discussed in this chapter. This chapter contains two case studies, the first is about moral residue in the global south and the second is about the ethics of empowerment.

Chapter 4 explores some of the main ethical considerations, tensions and challenges in health promotion practice. Within the chapter, the fundamental questions of whether aspects of health promotion practice are indeed ethical and may even contradict health promotion's key aim of improving health and reducing inequalities and social injustice are discussed. Drawing on debates such as those introduced by Guttman (2017), the chapter considers a range of questions such as 'Does health promotion actually promote health?', 'Who benefits from health promotion?' and 'Who are the winners and losers in health promotion?'. It concludes with a discussion about whether an ethical code of practice, frequently discussed by some, is necessary in order to provide an ethical framework for health promotion practice. This chapter includes two case studies, one about ethics and exclusion, and the other about ideologies of individualisation in the COVID-19 pandemic.

Chapter 5 discusses ethics as they are related to, and applied within, health promotion research. Starting with an examination of ethical principles as they apply to research studies and comparing them to health promotion ethics, this chapter then considers a broad range of ethical issues for health promotion researchers. Ethical approval processes and general ethical principles are critically discussed, to make a case for using situated ethical practices. By exploring research studies that work *with* people, rather than having data collection done on or to people, the links between health promotion as a discipline and research work that intends to affect social change will be discussed. The chapter discusses participatory, creative and inclusive methods of research as well as methods that privilege people's voices and experiences such as qualitative approaches to research. It considers the power dynamic in the research relationship and how this can be addressed. This chapter contains two case studies, one on indigenous research methods and ethics, and the other on ethical feminist research for social change.

Chapter 6 follows nicely from the previous one on ethical health promotion research in that it considers ethical evaluation as well as the ethical creation, and use of, evidence. As Green et al. (2019) state, ethics and evidence in health promotion are inextricably linked. The chapter considers some of the challenges in decision-making in evaluation, how we decide to evaluate and when, what measures are used to determine success, and what counts as evidence, and why. As well as unpicking ethical challenges with the evaluation process, the chapter also discusses the ethical considerations surrounding the use of appropriate evidence to make decisions about what works to promote health. Two case studies support the discussion in this chapter, one about evaluating the impact of a school gardening project on children's consumption of fruit and vegetables in the United Kingdom, and the other about community-based social innovation in Japan.

Finally, *Chapter 7* considers what an ethical future in health promotion might look like. This chapter picks up on the main themes presented in the previous six chapters and has two distinct halves. In the first half of the chapter, codes of ethics in health promotion are discussed, drawing on some existing frameworks and guidelines for health promotion practice. The chapter reflects on how ethical values and principles underpin these, and considers how they might be further developed for best practice. The latter half of this chapter covers issues of sustainability, taking into account the sustainability of health promotion and sustainability in relation to planetary health, and what it means to work ethically in relation to these. The chapter discusses the collective responsibility that those working in health promotion have to work in ethically sustainable ways to promote health. The chapter contains two case studies, one about food insecurity in Australia and the other about universal basic income.

It has been our pleasure to write this book and we hope you not only enjoy reading it but that it encourages you to think about ethics in health promotion. There are no easy answers to any of the questions and challenges we raise in this book but perhaps this it is one small step forward in the right direction – promoting equity, empowerment and social justice.

References

Beauchamp, T.L. and Childress, J.F. (2019) *Principles of Biomedical Ethics*. 8th Edn. Oxford, Oxford University Press.

Bunton, R. and Macdonald, G. (2004) Introduction. In: Bunton, R. and Macdonald, G. (Eds.), *Health Promotion: Disciplines, Diversity and Developments*. 2nd Edn. London, Routledge.

Green, J., Cross, R., Woodall, J. and Tones, K. (2019) *Health Promotion: Planning and Strategies*. 5th Edn. London, Sage.

Gregg, J. and O'Hara, L. (2007) Values and principles evident in current health promotion practice. *Health Promotion Journal of Australia*, 18 (1), 7–11.

Guttman, N. (2017) *Ethical Issues in Health Promotion and Communication Interventions*. Oxford Research Encyclopaedias: Communication. Oxford, Oxford University Press.

Sindall, C. (2002) Does health promotion need a code of ethics? *Health Promotion International*, 17 (3), 201–203.

1 Introduction to health promotion

Introduction

This chapter provides an introduction to health promotion as we, the authors, view it. It sets the context for the rest of this book, the basis from which we will consider ethics in health promotion. Those who are relatively new to health promotion should gain a good sense of what health promotion is about from this chapter and it should also serve as a useful reminder to those who already have some understanding of what health promotion is. The chapter details our perspective on health promotion and sets out how we see health promotion as distinct from, although part of, broader public health. We will discuss the three core values of health promotion starting with empowerment and equity. A discussion about the social determinants of health, which are central to the concerns of health promotion, leads into the consideration of the third core value, social justice. Key principles of health promotion are also introduced and discussed throughout the chapter. Finally, individual and structural approaches to health promotion are considered. The chapter contains two relevant case studies, one about health inequalities in the United States and the other about global road traffic injury.

By the end of this chapter, the reader should be able to:

- Understand and appreciate what health promotion is about;
- Identify and describe the core values and principles of health promotion and what sets health promotion apart from broader public health;
- Understand what social justice, equity and empowerment are and appreciate why they are central to health promotion;
- Understand the role social determinants play in the creation of health and how social justice is vital in tackling these;
- Critically appreciate the differences between individual and structural approaches to health promotion.

DOI: 10.4324/9781003308317-1

What is health promotion?

It is important to ascertain what we mean by the term 'health promotion' at the outset. Most texts start with an exploration of what 'health' is in order to provide a foundation for thinking about what it means to promote health; however, we will not be doing that here. Suffice to say that it is notable that there is no agreed definition of health in the literature. There is, however, general agreement that health is a highly complex, contextual and subjective phenomenon. As Woodall and Cross (2022) point out, 'health means different things to different people at different times in different contexts' (p. 7). We are not going to offer a definition of health here either, but it is important to point out that we perceive health to be of high value and as something that is not only desirable for all but also attainable for everyone under the right circumstances.

Different people will also have different understandings of what health promotion is about. The general consensus would be that it is concerned with promoting health, for example, maximising health gain or supporting the best possible health experience and outcomes. Some might conflate health education with health promotion; however, there are differences between the two (Whitehead, 2018). Likewise, some might conflate public health with health promotion but again, we perceive that these are not one and the same. In this chapter, we make a conceptual argument for why we see health promotion as a distinct area of practice, underpinned by an important and definable set of values and principles. These values and principles provide a fundamental guide for ethics and ethical decision-making in the health promotion field.

There is a limit to what an individual can do to promote their own health and the actions they can undertake for better health outcomes given that health is impacted upon by many diverse and complex factors. We will consider this later in the chapter in relation to the social determinants of health. At the outset, however, we will discuss the distinctions between health promotion and health education, and health promotion and public health. Before you read any further, please undertake Reflection on Practice 1.1.

Health promotion and health education

We concur with the perspective of authors like Sassen (2018), Gelius and Rütten (2018) and Whitehead (2018) who argue that health education is an important, necessary and complementary component of health promotion. Health education is distinct because of its focus on educating individuals in order to promote behaviour change; however, health promotion is much broader than that and encompasses many more types of activity at different levels from the micro level of individual lifestyles to the macro levels of policy and environment. Health education is largely

Reflection on Practice 1.1: Definitions

As discussed in this chapter, different terms have different meanings for different people. Take some time out to think about what the following terms mean to you:

• Health
• Health education
• Public health
• Health promotion

You might want to make some notes on each, or even try to come up with your own definition for these terms. Refer to these as you engage with the rest of the chapter content and reflect on the ways in which your ideas cohere or conflict with those that are presented.

concerned with preventative action whereas health promotion challenges the rather narrow focus on individual behaviour that health education supports and encompasses a much more comprehensive examination of the multiple, multi-level, interacting factors that influence health and health outcomes (Green et al., this volume; Wills, 2023). As Warwick-Booth et al. (2021) argue, '[health promotion's] ideological basis necessitates a move away from focusing at the individual level' (p. 281) and places the focus on the broader determinants of health instead. Thompson (2023) defines health education as 'informing and raising awareness of health issues', and views it as 'a vital first step' in promoting health (p. 8); however, as Wild and McGrath (2019) argue, it is not enough to simply give someone information. That alone will not have an impact on their health; people have to be able to act on that information and many factors will influence their ability to do so. Hence, the underpinning assumption of health education, that increased knowledge and awareness will result in changes in attitudes and behavioural attitudes, is flawed. The circumstances that we live our lives in will either constrain or provide opportunity for us to respond to health education information.

Health promotion can also be viewed as operating at the meso (community) and macro levels (regional/national/global) whilst health education is exclusive to the micro (individual) level (Pueyo-Garrigues and Armayor, 2023). Health promotion emerged as a distinct area in the 1980s as the limits of health education approaches began to be better appreciated in the context of the socio-economic factors that influence health and result in significant inequalities in health experience and outcomes (Hubley et al., 2021). Whilst health education approaches can lead to victim-blaming due to the reductionist emphasis on individual lifestyles and behaviours, health promotion diverts attention instead to the wider content in which those lifestyles and behaviours play out – the social determinants of health. It was in this context that the Ottawa Charter (World Health Organization [WHO], 1986), the cornerstone of contemporary health promotion, came into being which will be discussed in more detail later in this chapter.

Health promotion and public health

Thompson (2023) describes health promotion as 'an important arm of public health practice' (p. 7) explaining how it emerged as a defined area of practice quite recently (towards the end of the twentieth century) as compared with public health whose origins can be traced back for centuries. Many of the principles underpinning public health practice are the same as, or aligned with, those that underpin health promotion. For some people, there is little distinction between the two fields. For the purposes of this book, however, we view health promotion as an important facet of public health but distinctive in nature. Whilst public health's values are more aligned with paternalism (telling people *what to do* or doing things *for* them) health promotion is more about working *with* people. Public health is more concerned with health protection and health promotion is more concerned with advocacy, enabling and mediation as outlined in the Ottawa Charter (WHO, 1986) – see later discussion in this chapter for further details.

Like public health, health promotion is a multi-disciplinary activity and many people in different roles will have health promotion as a key part of their job (Hubley et al., 2021). Whilst public health is more medically focused in many ways, and therefore more aligned with a *biomedical* model of health, health promotion aligns more with a *social* model of health that better recognises the complexity of health. See Table 1.1 for a brief comparison between the (bio)medical model of health and the social model of health which underscores some of the key differences between public health and health promotion.

So far, we have discussed the distinctions between health promotion as compared with health education and public health. We now consider what health promotion *is* rather than what it is not. Health promotion is fundamentally about change for better health, whether that is change at an individual level (in behaviour) or in the conditions that create health such as our physical, social, political and economic environments. Health promotion is understood as a distinct disciplinary area that draws on other feeder disciplines such as psychology, sociology, epidemiology, policy, economics, communication and education (Bunton and Macdonald, 2002). Health promotion might also be conceived as a 'process or way of working that seeks to empower individuals and

Table 1.1 A comparison of the (bio)medical model of health and the social
model of health

(Bio)Medical model of health	Social model of health
Negative view of health	Positive view of health
Ill-health needs expert intervention	Ill-health requires collective intervention
Reductionist	Inclusive
Narrow understanding of health – health is defined as the absence of disease or illness	Broad understanding of health – health is socially constructed, subjectively experienced and multidimensional
Ill-health is caused by biological disruption	Ill-health is caused by social disruption
Emphasises personal responsibility for health	Emphasises collective, social responsibility for health
Focuses on individual behaviour change	Focuses on social change
Forms the basis of scientific healthcare systems	Forms the basis of traditional and alternative healthcare systems

Source: Cross et al. (2021, p. 9).

groups by valuing their experience and enabling them to address their
own needs' (Wills, 2023, p. 56). In keeping with this, other people view
health promotion as an inclusive social activity rather than the exclusive
activities of health professionals and experts (Pueyo-Garrigues and Armayor, 2023). Health promotion is also concerned with collective action
and can therefore be viewed as a social enterprise. Kickbusch (1986),
therefore, envisaged health promotion as being positive and dynamic.
Health promotion is also commonly described as an 'umbrella term'
(Scriven, 2017, p. 17) meaning that it covers a wide range of activities
or strategies that are intended to impact on the wider determinants of
health and that 'aim to facilitate people to achieve a full and healthy life'
(Evans et al. 2017, p. 13).

The WHO's definition of health promotion as laid out in the Ottawa
Charter (WHO, 1986) is well rehearsed (see Box 1.1) and provides the basis
for contemporary understandings of health promotion. Later refinements
to the nature of health promotion have resulted in the understanding that
it is a socio-political process which is intended to influence the social, political, environmental and economic determinants of health (WHO, 2012).

The Ottawa Charter (WHO, 1986) has been hugely influential in the
development of the global health promotion agenda since it emerged
from the first international conference on health promotion. The charter
set out five action areas that still guide practice today as follows:

1 Build healthy public policy;
2 Create supportive environments for health;

Box 1.1   Classic definition of health promotion (WHO, 1986)

Health promotion is the process of enabling people to increase control over the determinants of health, and thereby improve their health. To reach a state of complete physical, mental and social wellbeing, an individual or group must be able to identify and to realise ambitions, to satisfy needs, and to change or cope with the environment. Health is, therefore, seen as a resource for everyday life, not the objective of living. Health is a positive concept emphasising social and personal resources, as well as physical capabilities. Therefore, health promotion is not just the responsibility of the health sector but goes beyond healthy lifestyles to wellbeing.

---

3   Strengthen community action for health;
4   Develop personal skills;
5   Re-orient health services.

In addition, the Ottawa Charter proposed three core strategies for achieving effectiveness in the five action areas detailed above – advocating, enabling and mediating. See Box 1.2 for details.

Key values and principles in health promotion

Green et al. (2019) point to two major goals of health promotion that we uphold as key values – empowerment and equity – both of which are concerned with enabling people to gain more control over their health (as espoused in the WHO's definition – see Box 1.1). We now consider each of these briefly in turn.

Empowerment

The WHO's (1986) classic definition of health promotion (see Box 1.1) emphasises one of the most important values of health promotion – empowerment. Health promotion, as conceived by the WHO and others, is about empowering people to have more control over the things in their lives that affect their health (Scriven, 2017). As Cross et al. (2021) argue, health promotion is about putting 'people at the centre', empowering people and 'challenging the social structure' (p. 24). The WHO's (1986) definition highlights the need for people to be in control

Box 1.2 The Ottawa Charter's (WHO, 1986) three core health strategies for health promotion

Advocate - Good health is a major resource for social, economic and personal development and an important dimension of quality of life. Political, economic, social, cultural, environmental, behavioural and biological factors can all favour health or be harmful to it. Health promotion action aims at making these conditions favourable through advocacy for health.

Enable - Health promotion focuses on achieving equity in health. Health promotion action aims at reducing differences in current health status and ensuring equal opportunities and resources to enable all people to achieve their fullest health potential. This includes a secure foundation in a support environment, access to information, life skills and opportunities for making healthy choices. People cannot achieve their fullest health potential unless they are able to take control of those things which determine their health. This must apply equally to women and men.

Mediate - The prerequisites and prospects for health cannot be ensured by the health sector alone. More importantly, health promotion demands coordinated action by all concerned: by governments, by health and other social and economic sectors, by nongovernmental and voluntary organisation, by local authorities, by industry and by the media. People in all walks of life are involved as individuals, families and communities. Professional and social groups and health personnel have a major responsibility to mediate between differing interests in society for the pursuit of health.

Source: who.int/teams/health-promotion/enhanced-wellbeing/first-global-conference

of the things that influence their health. This means that people need a certain amount of power over their lives and what happens to them. However, many people do not have that level of power. Power is, therefore, regarded as a key determinant of health (Wills, 2023). Empowerment is viewed in health promotion as the key to better health and is fore fronted in the WHO's agenda for health promotion as evidenced in the documents, declarations and charters that have resulted from the various international conferences on health promotion that have taken place since the first one in Ottawa, Canada. The tenth most recent conference took place virtually in December 2021 and was hosted from Geneva, Switzerland. This conference focused on wellbeing, planetary health, and sustainability and again re-emphasised the importance of enabling people to take control over their health and lives (WHO, 2021).

Like health, there is no agreed definition of empowerment in the wider literature; however, we perceive it to be about people being able to have a say in what happens to them, having the capacity to make changes to their lives and having the opportunity to do so. Clearly this is not the case for everyone as power is not evenly distributed throughout societies (Cross et al., 2021). Health promotion aims to redress that imbalance for the benefit of everyone. There are some debates about whether empowerment is a process or an outcome or a combination of both; however, Green et al. (2019) argue that, generally, in health promotion, empowerment is viewed as a process of enabling people who lack power to gain a greater degree of control over their lives, that is become more powerful. But empowerment is not just about enabling individuals to have greater control over what happens to them, it also operates at the macro level – in communities, organisations and institutions (Laverack, 2006). There are also distinctions in the literature between individual empowerment and community empowerment. Whilst individual empowerment is concerned with concepts such as self-efficacy, self-esteem, control and personal agency, community empowerment is where people come together to create change for social good (Woodall et al., 2010). Both are linked of course – communities are made up of individuals after all. Empowerment, as a concept, is not without criticism and we will unpick some of the ethical challenges concerned with this value later in this book in Chapter 3.

Equity

Equity is another core value in health promotion. It is about fairness. Inequity is, therefore, a lack of fairness. The WHO (1998) states that equity in health means that people's needs guide the distribution of opportunities for wellbeing. The link with empowerment is therefore clear here. Green et al. (2019) argue that the achievement of equity in health is a major goal of health promotion. Equity is another of the key themes that run through the WHO's health promotion agenda which is primarily concerned with reducing the gap in health inequalities. Equity is one of the fundamental conditions and resources for health identified by the WHO (2009) alongside peace, shelter, education, food, income, a stable eco-system, sustainable resources and social justice. Woodall and Cross (2022) state that equity is 'a judgement on who is more or less deserving of support based on their social circumstances or conditions of living' (p. 82). Health promotion is therefore concerned with redressing the imbalance of power and health potential for everyone focusing on those with greatest need. This is therefore about fairness in resource allocation, fairness in access to health services and fairness in opportunity for health gain. In addition to the three core values that we are presenting in this chapter health promotion aligns itself with a set of principles. Box 1.3 outlines these in detail.

Box 1.3   Health promotion principles

1 Health promotion involves the population as a whole in the context of their everyday life, rather than focusing on people at risk for specific diseases. It enables people to take control over, and responsibility for, their health as an important component of everyday life – both as spontaneous and organised action for health. This requires full and continuing access to information about health and how it might be sought for by all the population, using, therefore, all dissemination methods available.

2 Health promotion is directed towards action on the determinants or causes of health. Health promotion, therefore, requires a close cooperation of sectors beyond health services, reflecting the diversity of conditions that influence health. Government, at both local and national levels, has a unique responsibility to at appropriately and in a timely way to ensure that the 'total' environment, which is beyond the control of individuals and groups, is conducive to health.

3 Health promotion combines diverse, but complementary, methods or approaches, including communication, education, legislation, fiscal measures, organisational change, community development and spontaneous local activities against health hazards.

4 Health promotion aims particularly at effective and concrete public participation. This focus requires the further development of problem-defining and decision-making life skills both individually and collectively.

5 Whilst health promotion is basically an activity in the health and social fields, and not a medical service, health professionals – particularly in primary healthcare – have an important role in nurturing and enabling health promotion. Health professionals should work towards developing their special contributions in education and health advocacy.

Source: WHO (2009, pp. 29–30)

These principles of health promotion underpin practice in the field and are ideologically informed by the values under discussion in this chapter. As well as the two fundamental values of empowerment and equity that we have discussed so far, research by Tilford et al. (2003) showed that people working in health promotion also identified a holistic view of health, equality, autonomy and justice or fairness as core values. Later in this chapter, we take up the latter in our discussion about the third key value we espouse – social justice – but first we turn the focus onto the social determinants of health.

Focusing on the social determinants of health

Before you read any further, undertake Reflection on Practice 1.2.

When we conceive of health promotion as recognising the central importance of wider influences on health (outside of the individual person), we can appreciate how the primary focus of health promotion becomes about addressing these influences in order to create the conditions necessary for health to thrive (Green et al., 2019). This focus is often referred to as the *social* determinants of health, sometimes as the *wider* determinants of health. The social determinants of health are the various and varying economic and social factors that impact on health such as income, gender, social class, level of education, ethnicity, faith, etc. As Wills (2023, p. 17) argues, 'these differences are not natural but are created and maintained by social and economic policies and legislation'. Health promotion recognises that health is fundamentally determined by many different factors. Wider influences refer to not only to our physical environment but also our socio-cultural-political-economic-global environment. There are several different frameworks that offer an explanation for the

---

Reflection on Practice 1.2: What determines health?

Whilst we have stopped short of offering a definition of health in this chapter, you will have your own understanding about what health means to you. Given that understanding take some time to think about the factors that influence your own health and the health of those around you. Start by making a list and then try to group the factors in some way to make sense of the different types of determinants of health that you are aware of. Carrying out this activity should help you to further appreciate the complexity of health and the numerous factors that influence and determine it.

wider determinants of health. A classic model of health determinants is offered by Dahlgren and Whitehead (1991). In this model, the individual is nested in the middle where the influences on health that cannot be changed (such as our genetic inheritance and our age) are represented. Moving outwards in concentric half-circles through the layers of the 'rainbow' framework lifestyle factors, social and community networks, living conditions and general socio-economic conditions are accounted for. This model is widely used as a framework for understanding the determinants of health, but it is not without its criticisms. Authors have noted its simplicity, the lack of account of interactions between the different influences, and the neglect of political, commercial and global influences on health (Warwick-Booth et al., 2021). In their Health Map model, Barton and Grant (2006) extended the rainbow idea to include factors such as the natural environment (i.e. air, water, land and natural habitats), the global ecosystem (i.e. climate change and biodiversity) and the macro-economy, politics and global forces as a way of conceptualising the determinants of health and wellbeing. The WHO later commissioned work on the social determinants of health that resulted in a further framework developed by Solar and Irwin (2010) which tries to make sense of the number and complexity of factors that influence, impact on and determine health (Warwick-Booth and Cross, 2018). Solar and Irwin's (2010) framework brings together many different factors including psychosocial, political, ecological and economic determinants. It distinguishes between structural determinants of health such as socioeconomic status, and intermediary determinants of health such as material circumstances (see Solar and Irwin's (2010) discussion paper for more details about this).

We do not have to look far to appreciate that people do not experience health in the same way. Whether we measure health in terms of objective measures such as disease prevalence or life expectancy, or subjective measures such as happiness or wellbeing, there are huge disparities. These disparities exist both within countries and between countries and exist across different dimensions such as race, ethnicity, gender, sexual orientation, age, disability status, socio-economic status and geographic location (Baciu et al., 2017). Close inspection will reveal that a range of factors come into play. See Case Study 1.1 as an example.

Health inequalities result from a complex interaction of many different factors. The biomedical model, introduced earlier in this chapter, only accounts for health inequalities in terms of our genetic inheritance, our age and disease or injury. However, most health inequality is socially determined, that is the influences that lie largely outside of our individual bodies or personal control such as working conditions, public policy, environmental factors, housing, etc., impact on our health.

Case Study 1.1   Health inequalities in the United States

Almost without exception all nation states will have health inequalities. The United States is used here as an illustration as it has some of the starkest in-country health inequalities in the world.

In comparison with peer nations, the United States ranks lower in the three key indicators of overall population health – infant mortality, age-adjusted death rates and life expectancy. Quality and length of life also vary according to race and ethnicity. Minority status populations fair worse on a range of health indicators; people holding multiple minority statuses even more so. For example, LGBT persons who are also in an ethnic minority have worse health outcomes than white LGBT persons. In terms of health care, access to services and support is unequal. For example, minority status people are less likely to have health care cover or insurance. Health care services are under-utilised by certain sub-populations such as Asian immigrants. Income inequality is directly linked to health inequality. The gap between the most well-off and the least-well-off in the United States has increased over the past three decades. The most well-off can expect the longest average life expectancy. The impact of climate change is not felt equally by everyone. Vulnerable communities are disproportionally affected by adverse conditions such as extreme weather events.

Source: Baciu et al. (2017)

Health inequalities and COVID-19

As in other high-income countries the global COVID-19 pandemic exacerbated existing health inequalities in the United States. Deaths from COVID-19 among black Americans were almost twice as many as those of white Americans. Whilst black Americans make up approximately 13% of the US population, they accounted for 24% of the deaths from COVID-19. This is against a background of inequalities in chronic disease which show the same pattern – excess diagnosis and excess deaths. Maternal mortality rates are three or four times higher for black women as compared with white women.

Source: Hopkins-Tanne (2020)

Box 1.4   Explanations for health inequalities

1 As a consequence of *lifestyles* – health experience is linked to risky individual behaviours such as smoking, lack of physical activity, eating unhealthily, etc.;
2 As a consequence of the *life course* – early life circumstances and the cumulative impact of exposure to different hazards over the life course contribute to health inequalities;
3 As a consequence of *psychosocial factors* – factors such as social exclusion and marginalisation, social cohesion and 'status anxiety' cause health inequalities;
4 As a consequence of *material disadvantage* – health inequalities result from the unequal distribution of resources in society;
5 As a consequence of *limited healthcare* – restricted (or lack of) access to healthcare services results in health inequalities.

Source: Wills (2023, pp. 28–32)

As Wills (2023) argues, social forces are significant in the creation of health inequalities. We do not have the space to consider the different social forces that contribute to health inequalities here suffice to say that they are many and varied. Wills (2023) presents five explanations for the existence of health inequalities – see Box 1.4 for details.

Case Study 1.1 illustrates many of the explanations for health inequalities presented in Box 1.4. Many of these inequalities can be avoided. Clearly, avoidable health inequalities and inequity can be addressed through different means which brings us to the final of our three core values, social justice.

Social justice

The third core value that we subscribe to in health promotion is social justice. Any consideration of the social determinants of health will lead to the conclusion that an individual has relatively little control over the factors that influence their own health. Choosing to eat healthy food might not simply be a case of making the right choices or lacking necessary knowledge about a well-balanced diet but will often be influenced by what is available, how much things cost and what products are promoted through advertising, etc. These factors are not in the control of the individual but of the state. Health promotion is therefore concerned with what are called 'upstream determinants of health' (Green et al., 2019). It is the state (or government) that is responsible for these. Thus, health promotion is inherently political, and health becomes, as Green et al. (2019) argue, an issue of social justice. Health promotion emphasises social justice which means that everyone should be treated fairly and equitably regardless of any differences arising from gender, age, ethnicity, faith, class, level of education, etc. (Linsley and Roll, 2020).

Social justice is a central feature within health promotion with its attendant focus on tackling health inequalities and addressing the root causes of inequity. Policy is therefore also a key area within health promotion. Healthy public policy should enable supportive environments – environments in which health can thrive. The importance of both healthy public policy and supportive environments was emphasised in the Ottawa Charter (WHO, 1986). We do not have to look too far to find evidence of health inequality (see also Case Study 1.1). If we consider a rudimentary measure of health, such as life expectancy, we can quickly appreciate that the number of years someone can expect to live, on average, varies not just between countries but within countries too. A body of work led by Sir Michael Marmot shows that health inequalities are actually increasing rather than decreasing. The global coronavirus pandemic which began in late 2019 has further exacerbated health inequality (Marmot et al., 2020). In terms of social justice, 'health follows a social gradient and therefore support, and intervention, need to be proportionately focused on those with greatest need' (Hubley et al., 2021, p. 20). This is what constitutes fairness – focusing efforts where need is greatest in order to reduce the inequality gap. The fundamental links between social justice and equity are therefore evident.

Power has been acknowledged as a key determinant of health (Krieger, 2008; Wills, 2023) and is a very important concept in health promotion and social justice. As Cross et al. (2021) argue, this means questioning who has power and who does not, how power is exercised, and thinking about how societies might be organised in much fairer ways for the benefit of the relatively disadvantaged. In this regard social justice is also very much linked to empowerment. Indeed, Laverack (2006) argues that empowerment is all about tackling injustice. Issues concerning social justice lie outside of individual control and are influenced by the social determinants of health; health promotion is therefore about the creation of equal opportunities and resources to enable the greatest potential for full health (Linsley and Roll, 2020).

Individual and structural approaches to promoting health

There are different approaches to health promotion outlined in the wider literature. Douglas et al. (2007) offer a distinction between individual and structural approaches which is of value here and lends itself to a higher level appreciation of ethical issues in health promotion. Individual approaches are concerned with encouraging individual health behaviour change by educating and supporting people. Individual approaches for health promotion 'operate under the assumption that it is possible for people to make [significant] changes to their lives and to their health' (Woodall and Cross, 2022, p. 35). On the other hand, structuralist approaches address the wider determinants of health as discussed in the previous section of this chapter. Structuralist approaches to health promotion can be understood as any activity that changes the structures in societies in which lives are lived in order to positively impact on health outcomes (Woodall and Cross, 2022). Some people, such as Whitehead and Irvine (2010), would argue that health promotion is more wedded to the latter approach and health education to the former; however, as previously stated, for the purposes of this book we view health education as part of health promotion, a view that is supported by Sassen's (2018) definition of health promotion as an overarching concept which includes health promotion where health promotion is understood as an 'umbrella' term (Scriven, 2017) as noted earlier in this chapter.

Hubley et al. (2021) caution against a simple binary presentation of individual versus structuralist approaches to health promotion given the complexity of health promotion practice; however, this is a useful way of broadly conceptualising different types of approaches. Midha and Sullivan (1998) offer a helpful comparison between individual and structuralist approaches in health promotion. They observe that individualist approaches tend to be victim-blaming, have a negative concept of health, and locate health promotion as primarily a medical, educational activity whilst structuralist approaches blame the system, have a positive concept of health and locate health promotion as primarily a social, political and cultural activity. Clearly health education, as outlined earlier in this chapter, sits within individualist approaches to health promotion. Structuralist approaches, in contrast, challenge the distribution of power in social systems as well as the allocation of resources and access to support. Case Study 1.2 presents examples of individual and structural approaches applied to the global public health challenge of road traffic injury.

Health promotion is critical of the standpoint that poor health outcomes are simply a result of poor behaviour or personal choices (Cross et al., 2021). This is reflected in the recommendations that have resulted from the body of work led by Sir Michael Marmot, the Commission on the Social Determinants of Health, which include focusing on upstream influences on health including improving the conditions of everyday life, redistributing power, money and resources, and determining the extent of the problem as well as assessing the impact of action (WHO, 2008; Schrecker, 2019). Upstream approaches to health promotion come under the remit of structural approaches and are concerned with addressing

Case Study 1.2   Individual versus structural approaches to road traffic injury

Road traffic injury is a significant global health issue. According to the WHO (2022), road traffic injuries are the leading cause of death for children and young adults aged 5–29 years; approximately 1.3 million people die each year as a result of road traffic collisions; more than half of all road traffic deaths are among vulnerable road users; 93% of the world's fatalities on the roads occur in low- and middle-income countries, even though these countries have only approximately 60% of the world's vehicles; and it is estimated that between 20 and 50 million people suffer non-fatal injuries with many incurring a disability as a result of their injury.

Individual approaches

Individual approaches tend to be aimed at the road users themselves (drivers, passengers, pedestrians, cyclists, etc.). For example, educating people about safer driving practices, driver awareness training, warning people about the risks of driving under the influence of alcohol or other drugs, promoting the use of motorcycle and bicycle helmets, and educating children about road safety and cycling proficiency. Focus tends to be on five behavioural risk factors – speeding, drink-driving, failing to use helmets, failing to use seatbelts and failing to use child restraints (WHO, 2018).

Structural approaches

Structural approaches are concerned with creating safer roads and vehicles, for example imposing speed limits, creating safer roadsides, mandatory vehicle maintenance, rapid emergency responses in the event of collisions and improving post-collision care, separate cycle lanes, enforcing seatbelt laws, tackling unsafe road infrastructure such as potholes, providing adequate facilities for pedestrians, that is safe places to walk and cross roads, instigating traffic calming measures, providing traffic-free zones, vehicle manufacturing standards and regulations, effective traffic law enforcement. All of these strategies are the responsibility of the state.

the so-called 'causes of the causes' of ill-health (Marmot et al., 2020). These include things like poor housing, unemployment, lack of money, lack of education and so on (Cross et al., 2021).

Finally, it is worth mentioning ecological approaches to health promotion. As Barton and Grant's (2006) model of determinants of health illustrates (see earlier discussion in this chapter) individual behaviour always occurs within a broader context. Ecological approaches can 'offer an alternative perspective that incorporates both individualistic and structural approaches and may provide a more effective strategy in tacking health inequalities [seeking to] understand the interrelations among diverse personal and environmental factors to human health and illness' (Hubley et al., 2021, p. 24). Socio-ecological approaches to health promotion take into account the various factors that influence individual behaviour which always, and without exception, occurs within a broader context.

Summary

This chapter has outlined our position on health promotion as compared with two other key related areas of practice – health education and public health. We have discussed what we see as the three core values of health promotion – empowerment, equity and social justice – and outlined some of the key principles that underpin health promotion practice. The WHO's role in the global development of health promotion has been acknowledged and discussed, particularly in relation to the seminal Ottawa Charter (WHO, 1986). Appreciating the social determinants of health is fundamental to the promotion of health and there are different approaches that can be taken in order to maximise health gain. We have discussed this in relation to individual and structural approaches and we also briefly introduced ecological approaches to health promotion. The next chapter will discuss how and why ethics are a key concern for health promotion.

Key points

- Health promotion is distinct from health education and from public health set apart by a discrete set of values (empowerment, equity and social justice) and distinguished by the focus on a social model of health.
- Health promotion operates from a defined set of principles.
- Approaches to health promotion can be conceptualised as individual or structural; however, individual approaches to health promotion are more aligned with health education whilst structural approaches are more aligned with health promotion.

Further reading

Woodall, J. and Cross, R. (2022) *Essentials of Health Promotion*. London, Sage. This is an essential guide to anyone wanting to know more about health promotion. It addresses the following questions: What is health promotion? Why is it important? When should health promotion be used? Who does health promotion? Where does health promotion take place? and How is health promotion delivered?

This is a more advanced critical and theoretical read about health promotion. It offers a comprehensive foundation in health promotion helping readers to understand and appreciate the process of planning, implementing and assessing health promotion programmes in the real world.

References

Baciu, A., Negussie, Y., Geller, A. and Weinstein, J.N. (2017) *Communities in Action: Pathways to Health Equity*. Washington DC, National Academies Press (US).

Barton, H. and Grant, M. (2006) *The Determinants of Health and Well-Being in Our Neighbourhoods*. The Health Impacts of the Built Environment, Institute of Public Health Ireland.

Bunton, R. and Macdonald, G. (2002) *Health Promotion: Disciplines, Diversity and Developments*. 2nd Edn. London, Routledge.

Cross, R., Rowlands, S. and Foster, S. (2021) The foundations of health promotion. In: Cross, R., Warwick-Booth, L., Rowlands, S., Woodall, J., O'Neil, I. and Foster, S. (Eds.), *Health Promotion: Global Principles and Practice*. 2nd Edn. Wallingford, CABI.

Dahlgren, G. and Whitehead, M. (1991) *Policies and Strategies for Promoting Social Equity in Health*. Stockholm, Institute of Future Studies.

Douglas, J., Earle, S., Handsley, S., Jones, L., Lloyd, C.E. and Spurr, S. (2007) *A Reader in Promoting Public Health: Challenge and Controversy*. London, SAGE Publications.

Evans, D., Coutsaftiki, D. and Fathers, C.P. (2017) *Health Promotion and Public Health for Nursing Students*. 3rd Edn. London, Sage.

Gelius, P. and Rütten, A. (2018) Conceptualizing structural change in health promotion: Why we still need to know more about theory. *Health Promotion International*, 33 (4), 657–664. http://dx.doi.org/10.1093/heapro/dax006

Green, J., Cross, R., Woodall, J. and Tones, K. (2024) *Health Promotion: Planning and Strategies*. 5th Edn. London, Sage. [Due for publication in January 2024 and on schedule]

Hopkins-Tanne, J. (2020) Ending US health inequalities needs multiple approaches, panel says. *BMJ*, 369, m2459. http://dx.doi.org/10.1136/bmj.m2459

Hubley, J., Copeman, J. and Woodall, J. (2021) *Practical Health Promotion*. 3rd Edn. Cambridge, Polity.

Kickbusch, I. (1986) Introduction to the journal. *Health Promotion International*, 1 (1), 3–4. http://dx.doi.org/10.1093/heapro/1.1.3

Krieger, N. (2008) Proximal, distal and the politics of causation: What's level got to do with it? *American Journal of Public Health*, 98 (2), 221–230.

Laverack, G. (2006) Improving health outcomes through community empowerment: A review of the literature. *Journal of Health, Population and Nutrition*, 24, 113–120.

Linsley, P. and Roll, C. (2020) *Health Promotion for Nursing Students*. London, Sage.

Marmot, M., Allen, J., Boyce, T., Goldblatt, P. and Morrison, J. (2020) *Health Equity in England: The Marmot Review Ten Years On*. London, Institute of Health Equity.

Midha, A. and Sulliva, M. (1998) The need to redefine the practice of health promotion in the United Kingdom. *Health Policy*, 44 (1), 19–30.

Pueyo-Garrigues, M. and Armayor, N.C. (2023) Defining health promotion and health education. In: Cross, R. (Ed.), *Health Education and Health Promotion in Nursing*. London, Sage. [Due for publication in November 2023 and on schedule]

Sassen, B. (2018) *Nursing: Health Education and Improving Patient Self-Management*. Springer.

Schrecker, T. (2019) The Commission on Social Determinants of Health: Ten years on, a tale of a sinking Stone, or a promise yet unrealised? *Critical Public Health*, 29 (5), 610–615.

Scriven, A. (2017) *Promoting Health: A Practical Guide*. 7th Edn. London, Elsevier.

Solar, O. and Irwin, A. (2010) A conceptual framework for action on the social determinants of health. *Social Determinants of Health Discussion Paper 2* (Policy and Practice). Geneva, World Health Organization.

Thompson, S. (2023) *The Essential Guide to Public Health and Health Promotion*. 2nd Edn. London, Routledge.

Tilford, S., Green J. and Tones, K. (2003) *Values, Health Promotion and Public Health*. Leeds: Centre for Health Promotion Research, Leeds Metropolitan University.

Warwick-Booth, L. and Cross, R. (2018) *Global Health Studies: A Social Determinants Perspective*. Cambridge, Polity.

Warwick-Booth, L., Cross, R. and Lowcock, D. (2021) *Contemporary Health Studies: An Introduction*. 2nd Edn. Cambridge, Polity.

Whitehead, D. (2018) Exploring health promotion and health education in nursing. *Nursing Standard*, 33 (8), 38–44. http://dx.doi.org/10.7748/ns.2018.e11220

Whitehead, D. and Irvine, F. (2010) *Health Promotion & Health Education in Nursing: A Framework for Practice*. London, Palgrave Macmillan.

Wild, K. and McGrath, M. (2019) *Public Health and Health Promotion for Nurses at a Glance*. Oxford, John Wiley & Sons.

Wills, J. (2023) *Foundations for Health Promotion*. 5th Edn. London, Elsevier.

Woodall, J. and Cross, R. (2022) *Essentials of Health Promotion*. London, Sage.

Woodall, J., Raine, G., South, J. and Warwick-Booth, L. (2010) *Empowerment & Health and Well-Being: Evidence Review*. Leeds, Centre for Health Promotion Research, Leeds Metropolitan University.

World Health Organization (WHO) (1986) The Ottawa charter for health promotion. *Health Promotion*, 1 (1), iii–v.

World Health Organization (WHO) (1998). *Health Promotion Glossary*. Geneva, World Health Organization.

World Health Organization (WHO) (2008). *Closing the Gap in a Generation: Health Equity Through Action on Social Determinants of Health.* Geneva, World Health Organization.

World Health Organization (WHO) (2009). *Milestones in Health Promotion: Statements from Global Conferences.* Geneva, World Health Organization.

World Health Organization (WHO). (2012). *Health education: Theoretical concepts, effective strategies and core competencies.* World Health Organization, Cairo. Retrieved from http://applications.emro.who.int/dsaf/EMRPUB_2012_EN_1362.pdf

World Health Organization (WHO). (2018). *Global Status Report on Road Safety 2018.* Geneva, WHO.

World Health Organization (WHO). (2021). *10th Global Conference on Health Promotion Charters a Path for Creating 'Well-Being Societies.* Geneva, World Health Organization.

World Health Organization (WHO). (2022). *Road traffic injuries: Key facts.* Retrieved from who.int/news-room/fact-sheets/detail/road-traffic-injuries

2 Ethics as a key concern for health promotion

Introduction

This chapter considers ethics as a key concern for health promotion generally as well as discussing some of the issues that health promotion faces from a philosophical perspective. It starts by considering what we understand by ethics. It moves on to a discussion about why ethics is a key component of health promotion and, subsequently, why it is therefore important to consider ethics in relation to health promotion. In doing so returns to the values and principles of health promotion that were outlined in the first chapter. Several ethical frameworks are presented and discussed including communitarian ethics. The chapter ends with an international case study on COVID-19.

By the end of this chapter the reader should be able to:

- Appreciate different ethical perspectives and the relevance of these to health promotion;
- Understand the values underpinning health promotion and how these may influence ethical considerations in theory and in practice;
- Understand and apply different ethical principles in health promotion;
- Appreciated the value of communitarian ethics for health promotion.

What do we understand by ethics?

There are many ways to understand what we mean by ethics. Different definitions exist in the wider literature as we will see; however, ethics are largely understood to be derived from our morals and values which, in turn, are influenced by ideology. Carter et al. (2011, p. 466) summarise ethics as 'the study of what should be done' whilst Hubley et al. (2021) define ethics as 'the study of morals, duties, values and virtues' (p. 29). They go on to state that 'values and ethical principles lead to moral imperatives', that is they lead us to make decisions or judgements about what should and should not be done. So, ethics can also be described

DOI: 10.4324/9781003308317-2

as 'the examination and discussion of the values underpinning conduct' (Duncan, 2021, p. 415). Cribb and Duncan (2002) offer a more detailed definition of ethics as follows:

> a disciplined attempt to (a) justify (or critique) particular values, or sets of values; and (b) to understand what kinds of conduct embody or promote those values. Put otherwise, it is about how we ought to live and act. It ranges from very abstract theoretical questions about the bases and nature of ethical judgement to more applied concerns with important social questions about, for example, human welfare, social justice, and our duties to other animals or the environment. (p. 217)

Ethics are socially constructed and evolve over time as our understandings about what it means to be human and live good lives change. As Wild and McGrath (2019, p. 97) state 'being fair and equitable will depend on what society feels is owed to others – it is therefore subjective and can be loaded with values and judgements'. Ethics are also influenced by morals. Morals can be understood as what Wills (2023, p. 84) defines as 'principles and beliefs about what is right and wrong, or good and bad'. These will also differ according to time, place and social context.

Ethics is about how we work and many professions therefore have codes of practice in place that provide guidelines for ethical practice – what should and should not be done, and under what circumstances. These link back to moral obligations and principles (Duncan, 2007). Ethical principles are also concerned with 'determining the priority given to health problems and the approaches to deal with those problems' (Issel, 2014, p. 92). For the purposes of the discussion in this book we take Duncan's (2007) position on ethics – that ethics involves questions about what we do and how we act as well as questions about value(s).

Health promotion values

Health promotion works from a set of values like any other profession or discipline. These values may or may not reflect the prevailing ideology of the society in which it is operating but the values of those promoting health will always be reflected in the decisions that are made about what is prioritised, what is done, how it is done, and how outcomes are determined and measured. Seedhouse (2009) argued that value judgements pervade all of health promotion and that health promotion is driven primarily by values rather than evidence of what works. Many values underpin health promotion including the right to participate, voluntarism, empowerment, self-determination and reflexivity. Community participation is also a key value, yet we do not always consider this, for example, in top-down approaches to promoting health. Central to the concerns of health promotion is how power operates and is dispersed or used. As discussed in Chapter 1, power is not evenly distributed throughout society which means that not everyone is in a position to exercise autonomy over their decisions and actions, this is particularly the case for disadvantaged, marginalised and vulnerable groups (Scriven, 2017). Health promotion is therefore also focused more on social and political changes rather than individual change. Last, but most importantly, health promotion, by definition, puts a high value on health and the attainment of it – 'the value of health for its own sake' (Duncan, 2021, p. 403). It is the certainty that health is of value that drives the promotion of health. This belief (or position) underpins everything that health promotion is about. However, not everyone has the same belief. People value different things for different reasons so we cannot assume that health is a normative value.

Ethical theory

Ethical theory arises from philosophy. Ethics is one of three branches of philosophy alongside *epistemology* ('enquiry into the nature and grounds of belief, experience and knowledge') and *metaphysics or logic* ('the study of the nature of being') (Duncan, 2021, p. 404). As stated earlier, ethics is concerned with what we do and how we act which, in turn, is based on what we consider to be of value or worth. Ethics is a sub-discipline of philosophy concerning 'values and the assessment of what is valuable' (Duncan, 2007, p. 147). This varies considerably depending on a range of factors including the context (and time) in which we live and our upbringing. For example, many people would hold the opinion that telling the truth and upholding the law are things of value; however, there are circumstances where not doing so could/would be justifiable such as when European citizens hid Jews from the Nazi regime. Whilst, arguably, this is an extreme example it is likely that you (the reader) will be able to think of many more.

Ethics has been described as 'a branch of philosophy that focuses on defining moral principles and what concepts and behaviours are morally right or wrong' (Wills, 2023, p. 84). There are generally considered to be three main schools of thought in ethical theory. First, ideas originating centuries ago with Aristotle about what it means to live a good life. Second, deontologist views concerned with the duty to act which were first developed by Kant who posited that we are obliged to take certain actions regardless of the outcome (i.e. tell the truth). Finally, there are consequentialist views which propose that we should, first and foremost,

Table 2.1 A brief overview of key ethical theory

Perspective	Key theorists	Key ideals
Aristotelianism or virtue theory	Aristotle (Greek)	Originating in Greek philosophy this perspective is concerned with what it means to live a good, moral, virtuous life. All people are considered to be of equal value.
Deontology	Immanuel Kant (German)	Based on the idea that we are obligated or duty-bound towards one another (the Greek word deonto means duty). There are rules we must follow; things we must or must not do. Recognises the notion of free well and that each of us has the capacity to act morally (or otherwise). Actions take place out of duty without regard for the consequences.
Consequentialism • Utilitarianism	John Stuart Mill (Scottish)	Concerned primarily with the consequences of taking action. Sometimes actions will have adverse effects. Therefore, action for action's sake is problematic. Whether an action is right or wrong depends on the outcome of it. An action is right or wrong depending on how much happiness results from it. The greater the resulting happiness, the more 'right' the action. Utilitarian theory is based on the premise of the greatest good for the greatest number.

Sources: Adapted from Cribb and Duncan (2002), Duncan (2021), Cross et al. (2021) and Wills (2023).

take into account the consequences of our actions. Consequentialism includes the Utilitarian view (the greatest good for the greatest number or the greatest happiness principle). Table 2.1 provides a more detailed overview these three perspectives.

A quick glance at Table 2.1 shows that ethical theory is dominated by male thinking from the global north. This is enough to conclude that there are many other ways of thinking about ethics that are not necessarily represented in general discussion, nor in the wider literature, which is worth bearing in mind. In fact, there isn't any agreed or universal position on ethics – it is a field full of disputes, challenges and arguments largely because it is conceptual rather than concrete. In short, this means that there are often no easy, straightforward answers. Judgements have to be made based on what we value or consider to be of worth. Nevertheless, there are a set of basic ethical principles that we can consider in relation to health promotion which can help guide the decisions we make and what we do. Namely then, 'ethics is concerned with making a series of judgements about what health means to the individual or community and about whether, when and how to intervene' (Evans et al., 2017, p. 20). It is concerned with what is acceptable and what is not. This will vary considerably according to several factors. As Wills (2023, p. 85) argues 'the purpose of ethical theory is not to provide answers, but to inform judgements and help people to work out whether certain courses of action are right or wrong'. Ethical theory and principles can therefore enable health promoters to decide what to do, and when and how to do it. After all, just because something *can* be done it does not mean that it *should* be done (Sindall, 2002).

Ethics as a key component of health promotion

Ethics is viewed as a secondary feeder discipline whose contribution to health promotion is perhaps less obvious than what Bunton and Macdonald (2002) refer to as 'primary feeder disciplines' (i.e. sociology, psychology, epidemiology, education, economics) which, they argued, have made more of a contribution to promotion theory and practice. So, whilst important, ethics has been seen as less so. However, we would argue that since Bunton and Macdonald conceptualised the idea of primary and secondary feeder disciplines 20 years ago ethics has a more vital role to play and perhaps should now be considered as a primary feeder discipline rather than a secondary one.

Ethics are taken into account in healthcare provision as a central concern. There is also a body of work around ethics in public health. In this book we are specifically considering ethics in relation to health promotion, as set out in Chapter 1. So, health promotion is viewed as distinct from public health but as a key part of it (Gardner, 2014). However, there are, inevitably, some overlaps between both healthcare and public health as many ethical concerns are relevant across all areas. We consider ethics to be of great relevance to health promotion, a key component if you like. This book is predicated on this idea. Carter et al. (2012, p. 1) argue that health promotion 'can be approached in two complementary ways: as a normative ideal and, and as a practice'. The normative ideal is concerned with how to achieve better health for everyone whilst the actual practice of health promotion is very broad ranging from implementing policy, to advocacy, to enabling individual behaviour change. Trying to promote people's health is predicated on assumptions of what better health is and what better health looks like for people. Once this is established health promotion is then concerned with how and when to intervene to try to achieve better health. Ethics therefore helps us to decide what to do and how.

To make things easier we might simply consider ethical concerns as 'dilemmas'. Many dilemmas arise in health promotion. These might be

Box 2.1   Ethical dilemmas in health promotion – some examples

- A community is experiencing ongoing issues accessing clean water which is causing frequent outbreaks of diarrheal disease in its young children. A health needs assessment takes place. When asked what the community think they need they ask for a football pitch;
- Despite meeting many times with their life coach and knowing the risks a client continues to smoke 20 cigarettes a day stating that their grandmother smoked all her life and lived to aged 92 years;
- A country rolls out a mandatory vaccination campaign for under 16-year-olds to tackle a highly infectious virus. The vaccination causes mild-to-moderate unpleasant reactions for 5% of the recipients and has 90% efficacy.

to do with how we allocate resources, who should benefit from intervention, what methods we use, how we carry out health promotion research, what we choose to evaluate when we are trying to determine what works to promote health and so on. See Box 2.1 for some examples.

Ethics is also about how we justify, and make sense of, our decisions and actions. The ethical dilemmas presented in Box 2.1 will have, no doubt, provoked some reactions in you (the reader). Those reactions will arise from the values that you hold – what you consider valuable. For instance, in the first example we might assume that the community values social health over physical health. In the second example the client is fully aware of the risks of smoking and continues to do so which is likely in conflict with the values of the life coach who has been trying to encourage them to quit. In the third example the majority of the recipients of the vaccination will benefit from it but a minority will likely experience some adverse reactions. This example raises issues about individual autonomy and rights. Case Study 2.1 raises many different types of ethical dilemma. As Cribb and Duncan (2002) argue, respect for autonomy is something that is not questioned in liberal individualist societies. Rather it is taken for granted as an accepted 'rule' within society. However, not everyone has the means to be autonomous and whether a person can exercise their autonomy will depend on a range of factors including the political climate and individual capacity for decision-making. As argued in Chapter 1, empowerment is a key component of health promotion and central to practice. Indeed, Green et al. (2019) state that being able to exercise the right to autonomy could

Case Study 2.1   Ethics and COVID-19

The global COVID-19 pandemic raised many ethical challenges. In efforts to promote (protect) population health many countries put into place a range of measures that caused ethical dilemmas for health promotion. 'From resource allocation and priority setting, physical distancing, public health surveillance, health-care workers' rights and obligations to conduct clinical trials, the COVID-19 pandemic presents serious ethical challenges' (World Health Organization[WHO], 2022a). We might also add mandatory requirements to wear face coverings and carry out regular self-testing.

Many of the measures put in place arguably infringed on human rights and removed individual autonomy in favour of the greater good for most of the population. Given that this is a global pandemic there is wide diversity between the social and cultural contexts of different countries which has been reflected in some of the local responses to the virus threat. In some countries mandatory vaccination has been put into place, in others the army was on the streets in the early days of lockdown making sure that people stayed at home. Whether these measures were adhered to was dependent on the specific social and cultural context and the prevailing political environment of particular countries or regions. What was ethically acceptable in one context wasn't necessarily so in another. In recognition of the complexity of the ethical issues that the response to COVID-19 provoked WHO set up an international Working Group on Ethics and COVID-19 in February 2020 to develop advice for Member States.

Mandatory vaccination

Vaccination is a very powerful form of health promotion. Some governments chose to make vaccination against COVID-19 mandatory whilst some opted for persuasive means to encourage people to comply. Mandating certain actions or behaviours is generally ethically justifiable for the protection of the public; however, this can cause tension with individual liberty and choice. WHO (2022b) proposed that the following ethical considerations need to be carefully thought through alongside other scientific, medical, legal and practical considerations as well as evolving evidence:

1 *Necessity and proportionality* – 'mandatory vaccination should be considered only it is necessary for, and proportionate to, the achievement of one or more important societal or institutional objectives' (i.e. the protection of population health);

2 *Sufficient evidence of vaccine safety* – 'data should be available that demonstrate the vaccine being mandated has been found to be sufficiently safe in the population for whom the vaccine is to be made mandatory';

3 *Sufficient evidence of vaccine efficacy and effectiveness* – 'data demonstrating that the vaccine is efficacious in the population for whom it is to be mandated and is an effective means of achieving the identified public health/societal/institutional objective should be available';

4 *Justice in access and availability* – 'as a condition for implementing a mandate, supply of the vaccine should be sufficient and reliable, and the populations that would be affected by the mandate should be able to easily access the vaccine without cost to them';

5 *Public trust* – 'policy makers have a duty to carefully consider the effect that mandating vaccination could have on public confidence and public trust, particularly on confidence in the scientific community and vaccination generally';

6 *Ethical process of decision-making* – 'policy makers have a duty to act in trustworthy way, which can be promoted through ethical processes of decision-making and communicating decisions to the public'.

These considerations reflect many of the theoretical ethical concepts that have been discussed within this chapter.

A further ethical issue concerning vaccines for COVID-19 was about access at a global level and illustrates huge disparities and inequities for health in terms of access. The European Union was criticised for betraying the global south in the delay of a temporary easing of intellectual property rights to allow for COVID-19 vaccinations to be produced on a greater scale. It was argued that this was a 'stark contrast to [the] original pledge [of the EU] that COVID-19 vaccines would become a global public good' (Corporate Europe Observatory, 2022).

be considered as the epitome of empowerment; however, other people's rights may be impinged upon in the process of an individual asserting their own rights. This illustrates how health promotion can be questioned in terms of process and outcomes (Wills, 2023). Box 2.2 presents some example questions. Take some time to consider these and then carry out Reflection on Practice 2.1.

Perhaps, more simply, we should end this section by considering ethics, as argued by Cribb and Duncan, as a 'form of academic enquiry into

---

Box 2.2   Ethical questions for health promotion

- Good health is a relative concept, so whose definition of health should take precedence? Is it ethical for a practitioner to persuade someone to adopt their perception of a healthier lifestyle?
- What means are justifiable to promote good health in the population? Should the interests of the majority always prevail?
- Since most ill health is avoidable, should those who knowingly adopt unhealthy behaviours be refused treatment?

Source: Wills (2023, p. 86)

Reflection on Practice 2.1

One of the questions posed by Wills (2023) (see Box 2.2) is as follows:

- What means are justifiable to promote good health in the population? Should the interests of the majority always prevail?

Take some time to consider this in more detail. This is about Utilitarian Theory. Can you think of any instances when the interests of the majority should outweigh the interests (rights) of the minority? Are there any circumstances in which the reverse situation is justifiable?

---

what is good and right, (that) helps to guide the way we ought to live' (Cribb and Duncan, 2002, p. 6). If we take this into account, then ethics in health promotion is about doing what is good and right. Of course, real life is a lot more complex than that, as is health promotion in all its forms. In addition, notions of 'good' and 'right' can be debated and contested, but that key principle should form the basis for action – doing what is good and right.

Why is it important to consider ethics in relation to health promotion?

It is important to consider ethics in health promotion because the nature of health promotion raises many ethical considerations that cannot be ignored. For example, the methods that are sometimes used may be called into account. Cross et al. (2017) point to a number of ways that health promotion operates that can be considered questionable such as the manipulation of emotions, the use of fear campaign and shock tactics, and of persuasion. Many factors determine what we do and do not do to promote health. Latterly economic considerations have become even more salient. Everything costs money so decisions about when, whether and how to intervene are also driven by economic priorities.

We need to consider several things in relation to ethical practice in health promotion. Chapter 4 will pick up on this discussion in more detail; however, it's worth considering this briefly here. Several questions can help guide ethical practice. Gardner (2014) offers three such questions:

- What are the ultimate goals? That is what 'good should it achieve'?
- How should this good be distributed?
- What means should be used to try to achieve and distribute this good?

Some of the answers to these types of questions can be found in how we think about responsibility for health. If we consider that health is the responsibility of the individual, then it stands to reason that individual autonomy should be more important than common good. If we consider that health is the responsibility of all (or of the state) then individual autonomy is of less importance. Case Study 2.1 highlights some of the tensions concerned with who is/should be responsible for health. As outlined in Chapter 1, health promotion views health as determined by social and structural factors rather than solely by individual behaviour or choices. There will always be a limit to the extent that an individual has responsibility for health and, therefore, autonomy over it.

Whilst we have been mostly considering the discipline or philosophy of ethics so far we need to recognise that what we are focusing on in this book is what is referred to as 'applied ethics'. In this respect we are thinking about ethics as applied to health promotion. As Cribb and Duncan (2002, p. 272) argue, this is about connecting 'the discipline of moral philosophy to areas of human concern and endeavour, including professional and occupational action'. Our area of 'human concerns and endeavour' is *health promotion.* 'As health promotion is tacitly concerned with creating a 'good' global society, with positive ramifications for health, it is inevitably bound up with ethical and moral questions. We are making judgments about what kind of society (world) we want to live in' (Cross et al., 2021, p. 163). Deciding what kind of society we want to be a part of comes down to ethical and moral considerations. For health promotion a 'good' society is one where everybody has access to health justice regardless of who they are. Cribb and Duncan (2002, p. 273) pose the (perhaps rhetorical question) 'What difficulty can there be in helping people stay healthy?'. Of course, there are many potential difficulties, especially when viewed from an ethical standpoint. In health promotion we can consider ethics on two levels – the practical level which is concerned with how health promotion is carried out (more on this in Chapter 4) and in relation to the big issues that health promotion is concerned with such as social justice, inequality and inequity.

Ethical frameworks

The simplest ethical framework is arguably based on the principle of 'do no harm'. The principle to avoid doing harm is enshrined in the Hippocratic Oath and is reflected in many health professionals' codes of conduct. Taylor et al. (2014) argue that the priority for health promotion must always be to do no harm. This could be considered a guiding principle for practice. The potential benefits and harms of all health promotion interventions should be carefully considered. This is the essence of ethical practice. Any breach would require 'a close examination of the multiple effects of (the) actions; some analysis of what are "good" and "bad" consequences; and how these difference kinds of consequences are to be identified and balanced together' (Cribb and Duncan, 2002, p. 275). However, the higher-order principle of health promotion, that the benefits of intervening outweigh any disadvantages, sometimes conflicts with other ethical principles (Berry, 2007). For example, enforcing seat-belt use through law takes away the individual autonomy to choose not to wear a seat-belt. Berry (2007, p. 110) therefore argues that we 'need to strike the right balance between allowing people to decide their own actions, whilst not allowing those actions to unduly inconvenience or damage the health of others'. This discussion will be picked up in more detail in Chapter 4.

In terms of biomedicine (or healthcare) Beauchamp and Childress (2019) offer a set of four ethical principles that are often applied to health promotion. These are autonomy, beneficence, non-maleficence and justice (see Box 2.3 for more details). The biomedical model does have some value in health promotion; however, whilst these four principles are a good starting point for health promotion there can often be some conflict between them. By way of example Sindall (2002) raises two questions – (1) under what circumstances would a health promotion perspective suggest that autonomy should be overridden in the interest of the greater good? and (2) what is health promotion's response when considerations of social justice conflict with rights or the maximisation of health? There will be many more questions like this when we drill down into the finer detail about what we do and why.

At times, the four principles might conflict with one another. For example, it is not always possible for everyone to exercise autonomy

---

Box 2.3   Four key principles of biomedical ethics

1 Autonomy (respect for persons and individual rights, acceptance of differences)
2 Beneficence (doing good, optimising benefits over problems, preventing harm)
3 Maleficence (not doing harm)
4 Justice (a fair distribution of benefits, risks and costs)

Source: Beauchamp and Childress (2019)

---

and their individual rights, especially when doing so puts other people at risk or undermines *their* right. Respecting people is a key concern in health promotion and this includes cultural sensitivity and respect for diversity. This is not just about autonomy it is about Aristotle's principle that everyone is of equal value irrespective of any differences they might have.

Justice is a key ethical principle for health promotion concerned as it is with issues of inequality and inequity. Justice is about fairness which is arguably an ethical principle itself. It is about the fair, equitable and appropriate treatment of everyone (Beauchamp and Childress, 2019). The underlying principle associated with justice is that 'everyone is valued equally and treated alike' (Wild and McGrath, 2019, p. 97). Justice is also linked to equity and equity is a key concern in health promotion. Both of these are about fairness which takes into consideration notions of need (who should benefit) which might also be based on 'some notion of merit' (Pitt and Lloyd, 2015, p. 296). Naidoo and Wills (2015, p. 436) define justice as 'fairness in terms of one or other (or more) or resource allocation (distributive justice), meeting natural rights (rights-based justice) and the law (legal justice)'. Many ethical issues will arise in health promotion relating to inequity in access and of resources, and in terms of what is prioritised (Schneider, 2017). Take some time out to do Reflection on Practice 2.2 which asks you to apply some of these ideas.

There are some challenges in applying a biomedical or healthcare understanding of ethics to health promotion's social model of health (as detailed in Chapter 1) given their concern with individual responsibility and behaviour change. So, whilst the four principles outlined by Beauchamp and Childress (2019) have value and are useful, we also need to think beyond these to develop an effective set of ethical principles for health promotion. As such Sindall (2002) asserts that the social model of

---

Reflection on Practice 2.2

Consider the different types of justice outlined by Naidoo and Wills (2015):

- Distributive justice;
- Rights-based justice;
- Legal justice.

How do these apply in the context/country in which you work or live? Think about this in relation to health and health promotion specifically. How are resources for health allocated? Is it fair? Equitable? Are some people's rights impinged upon in the pursuit of the health of the population? Are efforts to promote health carried out in fair ways under the law? Does the way that laws operate promote health for everyone?

---

health, as favoured by health promotion, requires a boarder framework than the biomedical one offered by Beauchamp and Childress (2019) and that the focus should be on the collective (or community) rather than the individual. The next section of this chapter on communitarian ethics will discuss this in more detail.

Gregg and O'Hara's (2007) theorising on health promotion considers three domains – philosophical, ethical and technical. These ideas will be discussed in more detail in Chapters 3–6; however, we will consider the ethical domain briefly here as it has direct relevance to the current discussion. According to Gregg and O'Hara (2007, p. 15) the ethical domain has four core values:

- 'Equity-based priority communities (the underpinning principle being that action should be prioritized for those with the most need)
- Equitable distribution of power (the underpinning principle being that power is equally distributed between all stakeholder);
- Ethical change processes (the underpinning principles being that change processes should enable active participation for those affected by an issue, should not impinge on people's personal autonomy, should be beneficial as a priority and, finally any potential harms should be considered and minimized);
- Evidence-based practice (the underpinning principle being that health promotion practice is based on evidence of need and effectiveness, and sound theoretical considerations'.

Cribb and Duncan (2002, p. 274) argue that 'fundamentally, the ethics of health promotion involves the careful examination of the authority or legitimacy of health promoters'. We could go further by suggesting that it is to do with the careful examination of health promotion itself – a very necessary thing. Health promotion is also concerned with respect for human rights and with sustainability. By sustainability we are referring to our *physical environment* which should take planetary health into account (we will pick up this discussion in more detail in Chapter 7) – and also the sustainability of health promotion. This brings to mind the adage 'give a person a fish and you feed them for a day, teach a person to fish and you feed them for life'. Ethical health promotion should be environmentally and socially sustainable.

Table 2.2 gives an overview of the main ethical frameworks and principles. Some of the content of this table echoes the ideas presented and discussed earlier in this chapter. Clearly there are some contradictions and conflicts between some of the principles here. For example, the principle underpinning utilitarian approaches to promoting health will necessarily undermine the rights of some individuals which is contrary to the principle of autonomy. Self-determination and choice would be void for a minority when utilitarian approaches are in effect. As Issel (2014, p. 106) argues, 'no single ethical approach to promoting health is inherently right or wrong'. The most commonly used approach is the

Table 2.2 Ethical frameworks and principles

Approach	Principle	Application to health promotion
Autonomy	Personal right to self-determination and choice	The choice of the individual choice takes priority and coercive measures are avoided.
Criticality (contractarian)	The worst off benefit the most	The greatest problem with the severest health risk is prioritised. The focus is on people at higher risk of ill-health.
Egalitarian	All people are of equal value; disparities are minimised	Everyone is treated equally with regards to respect, rights and opportunity. People deserve the same access to opportunities for better health.
Resource sensitive	Resources are scarce and finite	Decisions are made with cost-effectiveness as standard. Resources are allocated and expended for the greatest amount of health gain.
Utilitarian	The greatest good for the greatest number; the ends justify the means.	Collective benefits to whole populations or communities override individual choices or rights.

Source: Adapted from Issel (2014, p. 93).

utilitarian one; however, sometimes a combination of approaches is actually used depending on the issue and the context. The tension between the individual and the wider population is one of the main challenges in applying ethical principles in the promotion of health (Scriven, 2017). Where should the line be drawn between individual freedom and the health of the population? Does the means justify the ends?

Communitarian ethics

Carter et al. (2012) argue that the normative ideal of health promotion (basically the promotion of health for all) is underpinned by two broad ethical ideas – justice and community. Privileging the notion of community undermines some of the ethical ideas we have presented in this chapter as it means that the collective is valued over the individual so things like individual liberty and personal autonomy come second to the interests of the community as a whole. Health promotion's concern with issues such as social determinants of health, social justice and participation calls for an ethical framework that is broader than those that have been offered so far in this chapter which are largely derived from healthcare or biomedical ethics. Communitarianism is a theoretical perspective that takes into account the social and political dimensions neglected by the frameworks we have considered up to this point. It emphasises aspects such as social connectedness and de-emphasises the individual positioning them instead as part of a wider community (Sindall, 2002). As such it is much more aligned with the concerns of health promotion. The common good is taken into account, not just the rights of the individual.

Communitarian ethics 'moves beyond the principles derived from bioethics, to incorporate theories from social and political philosophy' (Sindall, 2002, p. 202). The premise is that people are part of a social context, rather than separate from it. As a result, the individual should not be considered as a single entity but as part of a (social) whole. Consequently, communitarianism promotes the notion of common good. Collective action is required in order to achieve common good. It is not, however, without its own (ethical) challenges for example, a question raised by Sindall (2002, p. 202) is 'what if community values conflict with other values, such as upholding the interests of minority groups?'. It is, of course, unethical to assume that everyone holds the same set of values (Scriven, 2017). In practice, we might often see situations where the concerns of health promoters are at odds with the concerns of the individual or community with whom they are working. As Stephens (2008, p. 37) argues 'an uncritical assumption that health promotion activities are an unalloyed virtue means that possible harmful effects are not considered. Apparently desirable objectives such as changing risky behaviours should be open to on-going questioning and examination'. With reference to research with First Nations communities in Canada, some health promotion scholars advocate the principle of an 'ethical space' where different world views are shared, valued and respected, and agreement about how to proceed is reached (Labonte et al., 2005). This idea, although originating from health promotion research, is congruent with a communitarian perspective that values the common good of society over the needs and rights of individuals. Finally, Wills (2023, p. 84) suggests that health promotion should be committed to the following:

- 'Respect for the rights, dignity, confidentiality and worth of individuals and groups;
- Prioritizing the needs of those experiencing poverty and social marginalization;
- Ensuring that health promotion action in beneficial and causes no harm;
- Being honest about what health promotion is, and what it can and cannot achieve;
- Building autonomy and self-respect as the basis for health promotion action; and
- Being accountable for the quality of one's own practice and taking responsibility for maintaining and improving one's knowledge and skills' (Abbasi et al., 2018; Dempsey et al., 2011 cited in Wills, 2023, p. 84).

Summary

You (the reader) will have noticed that this chapter has not set out to answer questions about ethics in health promotion, nor has it attempted to outline a specific and straightforward position. Instead, the aim was to raise several issues for consideration and to argue the case for why ethics are a key concern for health promotion. If anything, we would advocate that those working in health promotion in whatever area, and whatever level, need to be continually and critically reflexive about the values that drive their own practice and how these impact on what they do and how they act. As Sindall (2002, p. 201) argued 'in an increasingly pluralistic society the values from a single culture, religion or disciplinary perspective cannot be assumed, and it is necessary to work out our common values in the midst of diversity'.

The WHO (2022a) emphasises how health issues are becoming more and more complex resulting in an increasing number of ethical challenges. The same is true for health promotion, not least in view of the growing inequalities in health that exist within and between countries and in relation to issues of access to resources, equity, technology and supportive health policy. As Carter et al. (2012, p. 1) state, 'health promotion ethics is moral deliberation about health promotion and its practice'. This deliberation is (or should be) ongoing and iterative as understandings of health promotion and its outworking evolve and develop.

Key points

- Ethics is concerned with values and morals, and what is right and wrong which, in turns, influence how we act and what we do.
- Health promotion raises many ethical dilemmas that need to be reflected upon and addressed in practice; there are often no easy answers or solutions.
- Several ethical frameworks exist that offer utility for health promotion; however, communitarian ethics are most aligned with the values of health promotion.

Further reading

Beauchamp, T.L. and Childress, J.F. (2019) *Principles of Biomedical Ethics.* 8th Edn. Oxford: Oxford University Press.
This popular book provides a comprehensive account of the four ethical principles introduced in this chapter. Beauchamp and Childress's principles of biomedical ethics are widely cited in the literature on healthcare and public health ethics and applied in the health field.
Wills, J. (2023) Chapter 6: Ethical issues in health promotion. In: Wills, J. *Foundations of Health Promotion.* 5th Edn. London: Elsevier, pp. 84–96.
This is a very useful chapter that outlines the key ethical issues in health promotion. It should enable readers to further appreciate the ethical values and principles underpinning health promotion, to reflect on their own personal ethics, and to consider various ethical dilemmas that might arise in the promotion of health.

References

Abbasi, M., Majdzadeh, R., Zali, A., Karimi, A. and Akrami, F. (2018) The evolution of public health ethics frameworks: Systematic review of moral values and norms in public health policy. *Medicine Health Care Philosophy,* 21 (Sept. 3), 387–402.
Beauchamp, T.L. and Childress, J.F. (2019) *Principles of Biomedical Ethics.* 8th Edn. Oxford, Oxford University Press.
Berry, D. (2007) *Health Communication: Theory and Practice.* Maidenhead, Open University Press.
Bunton, R. and Macdonald, G. (Eds.) (2002) Introduction. In *Health Promotion: Disciplines, Diversity and Developments.* 2nd Edn. London: Routledge, pp. 1–8.

Carter, S.M., Cribb, A. and Allegrante, J.P. (2012) How to think about health promotion ethics. Public Health Reviews, 34 (1), 1–24.

Carter, S.M., Rychetnik, L., Lloyd, B., Kerridge, I.H., Baur, L., Bauman, A., Hooker, C. and Zask, A. (2011) Evidence, ethics, and values: A framework for health promotion. *American Journal of Public Health*, 101 (3), 465–472.

Corporate Europe Observatory. (2022) *TRIPS 'Waiver failure': EU betrayal of global south on vaccine access obscured by lack of transparency*. [Internet] Retrieved from https@//corporateeurope.org/en/2022/07/trips-waiver-failure-ue-betrayal-global-south-vaccine-access-obscured-lack-transparency

Cribb, A. and Duncan, P. (2002) Introducing ethics to health promotion. In: Bunton, R. and Macdonald, G. (Eds.), *Health Promotion: Disciplines, Diversity and Developments*. 2nd Edn. London: Routledge, pp. 271–283.

Cross, R., Davis, S. and O'Neil, I. (2017) *Health Communication: Theoretical and Critical Perspectives*. Cambridge, Polity.

Cross, R., Warwick-Booth, L., Rowlands, S., Woodall, J., O'Neil, I. and Foster, S. (2021) *Health Promotion: Global Principles and Practice*. 2nd Edn. Wallingford, CABI.

Dempsey, C., Battel-Kirk, B. and Barry, M. (2011) *The compHP core competencies framework for health promotion handbook*. Retrieved from https://www.iuphe.org/CompPH_Comptencies_Handbook.pdf

Duncan, P. (2007) *Critical Perspectives on Health*. Basingstoke, Palgrave Macmillan.

Duncan, P. (2021) Ethics and law. In: Naidoo, J. and Wills, J. (Eds.), *Health Studies: An Introduction*. 4th Edn. Basingstoke: Palgrave Macmillan, pp. 401–431.

Evans, D., Coutsaftiki, D. and Fathers, C.P. (2017) *Health Promotion and Public Health for Nursing Students*. London, Sage.

Gardner, J. (2014) Ethical issues in public health promotion. *SAJBL*, 7 (1), 30–33.

Green, J., Cross, R., Woodall, J. and Tones, K. (2019) *Health Promotion: Planning and Strategies*. 4th Edn. London, Sage.

Gregg, J. and O'Hara, L. (2007) The Red Lotus Health Promotion Model: A new Model for holistic, ecological and salutogenic Health Promotion practice. *Health Promotion Journal of Australia*, 18, 7–11.

Hubley, J., Copeman, J. and Woodall, J. (2021) *Practical Health Promotion*. 3rd Edn. Cambridge, Polity.

Issel, L.M. (2014) *Health Program Planning and Evaluation: A Practical, Systematic Approach for Community Health*. Burlington, MA, Jones & Bartlett Learning.

Labonte, R., Polanyi, M., Muhajarine, N., McIntosh, T. and Williams, A. (2005) Beyond the divides: Towards critical population health research. *Critical Public Health*, 15 (1), 5–17.

Naidoo, J. and Wills, J. (2015) *Health Studies: An Introduction*. 3rd Edn. London: Palgrave.

Pitt, B. and Lloyd, L. (2015) Social policy and health. In: Naidoo, J. and Wills, J. (Eds.), *Health Studies: An Introduction*. 3rd Edn. London: Palgrave, pp. 293–333.

Schneider, M. (2017) *Introduction to Public Health*. 5th Edn. Burlington MA, Jones & Bartlett Learning.

Scriven, A. (2017) *Ewles and Simnett's Promoting Health: A Practical Guide*. 7th Edn. London, Elsevier.

Seedhouse, D. (2009) *Ethics: The Heart of Health Care.* 3rd Edn. Chichester, John Wiley & Sons.

Sindall, C. (2002) Does health promotion need a code of ethics? *Health Promotion International,* 17 (3), 201–203.

Stephens, C. (2008) *Health Promotion: A Psychosocial Approach.* Maidenhead, Open University Press.

Taylor, J., O'Hara, L. and Barnes, M. (2014) Health promotion: A critical salutogenic science. *International Journal of Social Work and Human Services Practice,* 2, 283–290.

Wild, K. and McGrath, M. (2019) *Public Health and Health Promotion for Nurses at a Glance.* Oxford, Wiley.

Wills, J. (2023) *Foundations for Health Promotion.* 5th Edn. London, Elsevier.

World Health Organization (WHO). (2022a) *Global health ethics.* [Internet] Retrieved from www.who.int/health-topics/ethics-and-health

World Health Organization (WHO). (2022b) *COVID-19 and mandatory vaccination: Ethical considerations.* Policy Brief, 30 May 2022. Retrieved from WHO/2019-nCoV/Policy_brief/Mandatory_vaccination/20022.1

3   Key ethical debates in health promotion

Introduction

This chapter will consider some of the key ethical debates in health promotion and will discuss these with reference to case studies about moral injustices arising from interventions, as well as the ethics of empowerment approaches. Issues such as rights and responsibilities, agency and structure, the role of the state in health promotion, and the potential limits of autonomy will be considered. Using the Nuffield Ladder of Intervention as a framework for the discussion a number of questions will be considered such as when is it right to intervene? Is there a limit to personal choice? Does the greater good over-ride the right to personal freedom? There are a number of tensions in these debates that will be outlined and explored in this chapter. There will be an in-depth exploration of Nudge Theory and Choice Architecture – both of these 'methods' have been more recently lauded in behavioural science as a means of promoting health, but these raise a number of ethical issues worth exploring. Gregg and O'Hara's (2007) values and principles will also be considered in this chapter.

By the end of this chapter, the reader should be able to:

- Understand the key ethical debates taking place in health promotion;
- Identify and debate tensions found within these key ethical debates;
- Understand the importance of recognising and exploring ethical debates in the discipline of health promotion.

The role of the state in health promotion

The state or government is an important player in the policy-making process, with large scale remits of governance that influence and determine our health. Health policy is broad in scope, and covers efforts by the government to improve health, welfare and medical treatment.

DOI: 10.4324/9781003308317-3

It also includes policy interventions specifically focusing upon public health and health promotion. Given the range of determinants that influence health, and the weight of accompanying evidence about these, the contexts in which people live can either improve their health, or indeed make it worse (Warwick-Booth et al., 2021). Therefore, health promoters often call for health in all policies. Warwick-Booth et al. (2021) define health in all policies as attempts to tackle health and associated inequalities using all policy sectors, due to the recognition of the need for cross sector action in relation to the wider determinants of health arising from the economic, commercial, social and environmental contexts of people's lives. There have been many state-led public health interventions, which have improved health, through direct and indirect interventions (health in all policies), though these raise ethical questions. Furthermore, balancing individual rights versus their responsibilities as citizens of the state also raises debate. Policy makers increasingly call upon citizens to be more responsible in their health behaviours, for example by eating less unhealthy food, and taking more exercise – they are expected to behave as morally responsible agents. However, this is a more complex expectation than it initially seems, given that health choices take place in specific contexts which determine choice (Brown et al., 2019), therefore debates about the ethics of individual agency require critical analysis. Furthermore, the ethics of all health promotion policies require as some have historically caused injustice and harm. Box 3.1 provides

---

Case Study 3.1   Moral residue in the global south and its ethical implications

Ujewe (2018) discusses the moral residue left over from previous interventions in the global south which serve to limit progress in terms of global health. Though well intended some public health interventions, supported by a global community of policy makers and practitioners, have resulted in *'lingering feelings of anxiety, anger, blame or frustration ... among local populations where previous interventions ... have left traces of harm and/or exploitation.'* Ujewe (2018, p. 96). Little consideration has been given to how such moral residue affects contemporary health improvement approaches. Thus, there is a need to work in more ethical ways, creating harmony by understanding cultural contexts, and including the processes, resources and concerns of the communities in which interventions are being delivered. Ethical public health work in the global south needs to focus on holistic benefits for populations rather than just achieving goals, which may not even align with population health wants. Such approaches should consider the following:

- The ethical dilemmas and challenges faced by humanitarian relief workers, when working to tackle health crises;
- The moral and ethical experiences of those at the receiving end of global health actions, and the after-effects of these experiences;
- The intentions of funding agencies, researchers and health workers who are based in the global north? What too of more local power structures, and the intentions of their employees, including public health workers?

a case study of the ethical implications of historical health promotion interventions.

There are many more examples of ethical tensions underpinning health promotion interventions, highlighted by the Nuffield Bioethics Council (2007) (2007), through a ladder of interventions.

The Nuffield Ladder

Given that all interventions and measures to improve public health, lead to questions about the relationship between the state, and the individuals within it, as well as the ethics of such approaches, it is challenging to decide when it is right to intervene and in what circumstances individual choices should be limited, as well as when consent is required, compared to when it is not. The Nuffield Bioethics Council (2007, 2.22–2.26) suggests that individual consent is not always required, when interventions are not 'very intrusive' or 'prevent significant harm to others'; however, some interventions are more invasive. Ethical debates related to public health interventions are illustrated in Table 3.1.

As Table 3.1 shows, there are various levels of intervention, and at each of these, ethical questions can be posed. Griffiths and West (2015) argue that the ladder described in Table 3.1 is one-sided as it tends to view any intervention as a cost to personal autonomy, hence a more balanced view is needed, moving beyond examining just the two values of autonomy and welfare. Furthermore, Gray (2013) highlights the ways in which public health professionals and governments frequently disagree on effective interventions to improve public health, because of changing understandings of socio-political acceptability. Such disagreements are linked to values, evidence and the proportionality of the intervention in terms of its success versus its effect on people, and its financial cost.

Table 3.1 The Nuffield Ladder of potential interventions for government consideration

Possible action related to choice	Example of its application and associated ethical questions
Remove all choice	The use of national lockdowns in response to COVID-19 infection rates, intended to protect health raised ethical questions about potential harm to those who were least at risk, such as young people. Inequalities were also potentially made more severe for some individuals and groups from these policies (Frith, 2020). Cheung and Ip (2020) also highlight the ethical challenge of protecting physical health, whilst potentially leaving a legacy of mental health issues resulting from lockdown experiences.
Limit choices	Policy increasingly limits individual choices in relation to smoking, for example via smoking bans. These are intended to improve health, by reducing smoking rates as well as exposure to second-hand smoke. Evidence suggests that these objectives have been met to some extent, though full evaluation of their success is not possible for a number of years (Gagliani, 2019). However, van der Eijk and Porter (2013), discuss the ways in which pro-smoking advocates have referred to individuals rights to liberty, self-determination and privacy to make a case for them choosing to smoke. Ethical tensions are evident here when the state is attempting to protect life and health, yet limiting individual liberty.
Influence and guide choice through deterrents	Fiscal policy (concerned with taxation and spending) can be used to deter people's choices in various ways. For example, increasing taxation on unhealthy sugary drink options has been shown to reduce their consumption, leading to better longer term health outcomes including reductions in levels of diabetes (World Health Organization [WHO], 2017). WHO (2022) also highlights evidence to show that increasing tax on alcohol has life-saving effects, reducing deaths from a range non-communicable diseases. However, opponents of these approaches argue that they are illiberal and unethical as well as paternalistic, therefore they should be avoided as they remove choice (Goiana-da-Silva et al., 2020).
Influence and guide choice through rewards	This type of intervention, can also use fiscal policy but as mechanism to offer rewards to people. Ananthapavan et al. (2018) provide evidence about the effectiveness of using financial rewards to encourage obese people to lose weight. Offering payments encourages people to participate in interventions and reduces dropout rates. However, ethical questions remain about the impact of these approaches in the longer-term, the ways in which rewards coerce people and potentially increase inequalities (Halpern et al., 2009).

(Continued)

Table 3.1 (Continued)

Possible action related to choice	Example of its application and associated ethical questions
Influence and guide choice through changing policy	This type of intervention is about steering people through changing the options that are available to them. Nudge approaches based upon choice architecture fall within this category, and are discussed in depth later in this chapter. They can include steering people towards picking healthier food options, and nudging them to take more exercise (Nuffield Bioethics Council, 2007). Ethical questions about steering people at an unconscious level are frequently discussed in the literature: does 'guiding' people in such ways removes their liberty and freedom of choice (Rouyard et al., 2022)?
Encourage and enable choice	Interventions in this category encourage and enable healthier choices, for example, through the provision of public health services such as weight management, and stop smoking support. These are arguably more ethical in that they allow people to choose to opt into the services. However, critical analysis of weight loss services suggests that ethical challenges remain. For example, there may be gender differences linked to social norms about body image resulting in more harmful practices around weight loss for women and support services may cause moral distress to participants (Mills, 2023).
Information provision	In this approach, people are offered in information to support their health education, for example, about eating healthy or taking more exercise. This seems ethical at first glance given that information in simple terms can be heard, or ignored therefore, individuals retain their liberty to choose. However, Guttman (2017) argues that there may be vested interests at play in defining the information that is communicated and that appeals can be highly emotional. Ethical questions abound. Information provision is also not equitably heard across all social groups, thus attention needs to be paid to such exclusions.
Take no action and/or observe the situation	Policy makers can also choose to do nothing, and/or simply monitor a situation taking a precautionary stance. For example, employers may choose to do nothing to support the health and wellbeing of their workers, for fear of offending, demotivating or indeed alienating them. However, doing nothing could in itself be unethical, if working conditions lead to stress and other health problems such as postural injuries from sedentary working practices. Cavico and Mujtaba (2013) debate the ethics of wellness policies, and argue that it is more ethical for employers to support wellbeing than it is for them to take no action at all. Others (e.g. Kwoh 2013) argue that these approaches should not be used as they are unethically informed by employers motivations.

Source: Adapted from Nuffield Bioethics Council (2007).

Reflection on Practice 3.1: Balancing interventions against personal choice

The WHO (2023) recommends that adults should consume no more than 5 g of salt on a daily basis, suggesting that government policy should support this to improve health outcomes. Some countries are already drawing up policy actions to reduce salt in food production, focusing on the high levels of salt found in processed food such as sliced bread (Action on Salt, 2023) as well as considering banning the advertising of salty foods (Department of Health and Social Care, 2022). In the future some salty foods may also be banned from sale.

Using the following questions drawn from the Nuffield Ladder, reflect on your own views about the restriction of unhealthy salty food products:

1 Is it right to intervene in this issue?
2 Is there a limit to personal choice? Does this need to be adapted to each issue, and what considerations need to be also be made?
3 Does the greater good always over-ride the right to personal freedom?

Reflection 3.1 enables you to consider your own values in relation to dietary choice.

Braithwaite (2022) discusses the hypothetical implementation of policy to restrict salt intake, arguing that many public health professionals view this type of restriction as being akin to seatbelt laws, and so many are in favour. However, he argues that seatbelt legislation saves many lives, whereas salt restriction is likely to afford individuals only two weeks extra life, whilst reducing their wellbeing, if they find satisfaction from consuming salt. He also asks if salt restrictions may simply push individuals into consuming more fatty foods, arguing that population level interventions are wrongly assumed to be ethical before they have even been piloted to test their effectiveness. These debates have led to the use of policies which do not restrict population health choice, rather they attempt to steer people into healthier behaviours.

Nudge theory and choice architecture

The concept of 'nudge' has been used in UK and US policy approaches, attempting to promote healthier behaviours. Based on social marketing, this involves a range of approaches which aim to prod or gently change social and physical environments to make certain healthier behaviours more likely (Thaler and Sunstein, 2009). 'Nudge' is based on the idea that small changes in our immediate environment or context can 'nudge' (or encourage) us to behave in different ways and/or make different (i.e., healthier) choices (Loibl et al., 2018). Thaler and Sunstein (2009) argue that small changes can have a large impact on the way in which people behave and the choices that they make. The idea of nudge is essentially a mechanism to make whole populations change or modify their behaviour (Marteau et al., 2011), through choice architecture. 'Choice architecture' refers to the ways in which environments, contexts and situations can be altered to influence people's decision-making and therefore behaviour. Choice architects are those in roles holding *'responsibility for organizing the context in which people make decisions'* (Thaler and Sunstein, 2009, p. 3), and can therefore include health promoters. From a health promotion perspective, choice architecture is about altering environments so that people make healthier choices, without necessarily restricting their individual freedom (Cross et al., 2017). Based on behavioural economic approaches (Lodge and Wegrich, 2016), nudge and choice architecture work at an unconscious level for the most part (Marteau et al., 2011), and so their value is increasingly being seen in relation to food choices, as populations' diets tend to fall short of healthy recommendations. Ensaff (2021) argues that there is encouraging evidence on the effects of nudging populations towards healthier eating. Changing default choices on menu settings (salad rather than chips), placing unhealthy foods in different locations in shops (moving them away from where people queue) and reducing portion sizes on unhealthy options have been all been shown to be effective nudge strategies. Indeed, nudge strategies are already used effectively for commercial purposes such as in supermarket settings, to encourage healthier purchasing (Huitink et al., 2020).

Criticism of nudges have been wide-ranging, and there is minimal evidence of their effectiveness to improve health at a population, yet they appeal to policy makers because it is low cost and does not require legislation (Arno and Thomas, 2016). Ethical questions frequently arise in relation to evidence-based decision-making (see Chapter 6 for more discussion on this). Minimal state intervention is an ideological aspiration, which plots at a low level on the Nuffield Ladder of Intervention (Nuffield Bioethics Council, 2007, p. 128), moving focus away from the nanny state. Despite the appeal of the concept, the ethics of the approach requires much consideration. Nudging people parallels with the marketing approaches used by large companies, is individualistic, and Western in its origins. Marteau et al. (2011) argue, the strategy of nudge is one widely used by the advertising industry. As a result, *'subtle changes to the context or environment in which individuals make decisions may have powerful implications for behaviour change'* (Martin et al., 2020, p. 53). Box 3.1 summarises some of the key ethical debates about nudging for health promotion.

There are many ethical questions related to the use of nudge as an approach to promote health, and some of these relate to the balance between structure and agency; the extent to which individuals should

---

Box 3.1 Ethical debates about nudging for health promotion

- Nudge is unethical because it undermines the liberty of people and their freedom of choice, because their unconscious mind is being manipulated. If we are being nudged to behave in certain (healthier) ways and make decisions that we otherwise would not have made, then we simply are not free to do as we wish (Cross et al., 2020). Nudge-based approaches are manipulative, coercive and persuasive, which contradict the principles of health promotion practice, and align with nanny state approaches (Chriss, 2015) therefore using such an approach is unethical (Lin et al., 2017). Chapter 4 discusses how some health promotion interventions have been described as unethical.

- Do policy makers and health promoters know better than individuals about what they should be doing (Chriss, 2015), and how they should be behaving?

- Selinger and Whyte (2011, p. 92) argue that nudge techniques already exist, and that the more that these are applied in practice, '*the less we may be bothered by the incremental introduction of more controlling tactics*', which is a major ethical drawback.

- 'Nudging' people towards changing their behaviour assumes that those in power know that people want 'better health and longer life' (Hastings and Stead, 2006, p. 141). This is paternalistic, because it is trying to '*influence people's behaviour in order to ... make their lives healthier*' (Thaler and Sunstein, 2009, p. 5), irrespective of the rationale offered for this being legitimate.

- Nudge is ethically misaligned to the health promotion concept of empowerment, does nudge enable people to take control of their health and their lives, or instead is it a mechanism to remove control away from individuals (Cross et al., 2020)?

- Robinson (2020) also questions the use of nudge in the global south, where cultural differences may conflict with western ethical values. Furthermore, public support for nudge-based interventions varies according to country context, and evidence about them in lower income countries is lacking (Ledderer et al., 2020).

make their own decisions, versus the power of the state and its role in promoting health.

Health promotion: the interface between structure and agency?

Despite some government successes in promoting health, debates exist in relation of the responsibility of citizens, to promote their own health through individual agency. Decades of debate have taken place in the field of Sociology about how to define the concept of agency, as well as the extent to which structure and agency influence health. Giddens (1984, p. 9) suggests that *'Agency refers not to the intentions people have in doing things but to their capability of doing those things in the first place .... Agency concerns events of which an individual is the perpetrator, in the sense that the individual could, at any phase in a given sequence of conduct, have acted differently.'* Given that poverty and social inequality damage individuals' and communities' capacity for action, resulting in limited agency (Cross et al., 2020). Giddens (1984) proposed the theory of structuration, in which he recognised the inter-relationship and co-dependence between structure and agency. Structures are recognised in shaping individuals' practices and actions, but it remains the case that individuals' practices and actions also constitute and reproduce structures (Sibeon, 1999; Warwick-Booth, 2022).

Debates have long since existed about the extent of power within societal structures, compared to each person's agency, both impacting upon health to various extents. Dahlgren and Whitehead's (1991) model reflects the range of influences at play, and was later developed to include a global focus by Barton and Grant (2006). Cockerham (2007, p. 55) also asked *'Are the decisions people make with respect to food, exercise, smoking, and the like largely a matter of individual choice or are they principally moulded by structural variables such as social class position and gender?'* Weber long since made links between class position, economics and lifestyle (Cockerham et al., 1997). Bourdieu's (1984) concept of habitus demonstrated how life chances (structures) and predispositions determine and influence life choices. Bourdieu argued that whilst people choose their lifestyle they do not do this as freely as they think; instead, their choices are underpinned by their habitus, and rules that are appropriate to their social situation. Other theorists refer to social norms which guide and indeed bound individual choices, including those around health. Those who are economically better off are more able to make healthier choices (Marmot, 2017).

In light of all of this, health promotion as a discipline suggests that healthier choices can be achieved through health in all policies, as outlined earlier, as well as through the creation of supportive environments and settings in which the 'healthy choice' is the 'easy choice' (Kickbusch, 1986; Milio, 1986). Some health promotion scholars argue that the concept of 'free choice' is to an extent an illusion due to the way in which the wider structural environment plays a major role in our health-related choices (Tones, 1998; Green, 2004; Warwick-Booth, 2022). Health promotion therefore remains political (Tones, 1998) because the ethics of promoting health in such complex societal circumstances, remain tied to political viewpoints.

Health promotion is an inherently political enterprise with some of its most compelling critiques emanating from diametrically opposed political viewpoints which embrace collectivism or individualism (Davison and Davey Smith, 1995; Kelly and Charlton, 1995, Nettleton, 1995; Naidoo and Wills, 2009). For example, a left wing perspective would see disadvantaged groups having limited power and choice in affecting the determinants that influence their health. This perspective advocates for collective solutions and interventions aimed at social justice (a core principle of health promotion, discussed in Chapter 1) to reduce inequalities in health (Davison and Davey Smith, 1995). On the other hand, debates from the right make a case for the primacy of the individual and prioritise the notion of personal choice (Davison and Davey Smith, 1995). Irrespective of these theoretical differences, ethical questions remain about the use of choice to promote health in an unequal world. Box 3.2 offers some example ethical questions in relation to making healthier choices.

As Box 3.2 illustrates, there are many ethical questions about the promotion of choice. Despite these questions and ethical issues, it remains the case that health promoters frequently cite the importance of empowerment as an approach to facilitate individuals and communities taking control, making choices and challenging structural constraints (see Chapter 1). The concept is difficult to define (Woodall et al., 2012) and even harder to measure (Cross et al., 2017) yet is remains a fundamental tenet of health promotion practice, applied at both the individual and community level (Wallerstein, 1992). Individual empowerment is made up of a cluster of attributes which support the realisation of personal capacity, for example through confidence building, boosting self-esteem and enhancing personal skills (Thompson, 2007). Individual empowerment is where people have a relatively high degree of power and therefore greater potential for making choices (Tones and Tilford, 2001). Consequently empowered people often have better health given that they are more capable of making informed decisions about their life (Rodwell, 1996; Linhorst et al., 2002; Larsen and Manderson, 2009). Empowerment is therefore assumed to lead to healthier lifestyle choices (Bakhshi et al., 2017). Policy makers in the global north are increasingly focus on promoting the choice of a healthy lifestyle to citizens, arguing that they need to take responsibility, ignoring the differences that exist in

---

**Box 3.2   Ethical questions about the promotion
of choice in an unequal world**

- Do people have the right to choose not to be healthy? The
  ethics of making unhealthy choices is an interesting area. If
  I choose to smoke, eat unhealthy foods, and take no exercise
  then are my choices morally wrong? Where does blame lie for
  those making such choices, and why?
- If health promotion determines choices, then is it simply a
  form of health fascism (Downie et al., 1996). Gardner and
  Biko (2014) suggest that many health promotion strategies can
  be ethically problematic as choices are influenced by coercion,
  persuasion, manipulation and indeed deception.
- Are some choices more ethically challenging than others, and
  if so what does this mean for those making decisions? Cho
  et al. (2020) discuss patient choices in relation to health care,
  suggesting that choices related to end-of-life care, genetic testing and reproductive health are more ethically challenging. In
  exploring patient concerns, their research also highlighted the
  wider implications of choice, beyond the individual, into family contexts.
- Does offering people choice improve their wellbeing and enhance their freedoms? Do people want more choice? Is too
  much choice more of a burden? Schwartz and Cheek (2017)
  pose these questions, all of which are relevant to the ethics of
  offering choice through social policies.

---

capacity to choose due to structural inequalities (Marmot, 2017). This
has long been recognised in the literature (see Wallerstein, 1992). However, policy makers still tend to focus on lifestyle interventions without
considering the ethical implications of their actions, which has led to
some health promoters calling for more of a focus on community empowerment. This is seen by some as being more political and ethically
oriented in focus, intending to support the redistribution of resources,
challenging social injustice and oppression (Ward and Mullender, 1991;
Rissel, 1994), through community level action (Baum, 2003). However,
ethical tensions remain evident in health promotion practice, that draws
on empowerment approaches. Case Study 3.2 discusses some of these.

As Case Study 3.2 highlights, all public health and health promotion
principles can be debated. Furthermore, there are many health promotion approaches, aligning with different political positions, all of which

Case Study 3.2 The ethics of empowerment for health promotion

Tengland (2016) highlights the ethical dilemma associated with empowering some groups, which then might result in them increasing the power that they have over others. Furthermore, empowered people might also make unhealthy choices, or risk their health through engaging in potentially damaging activities such as extreme sports. Empowerment may also result in people realising that health is not the most important thing in their lives. Spencer (2015) draws attention to the unintended consequences of empowerment approaches, which raise ethical questions, and additionally result in outcomes that may not be considered positive in health promotion terms. She questions the idea that working with people's own health related concerns is an automatic route to empowerment. Braunack-Mayer and Louise (2008) also argue that community empowerment is ethically problematic. First, they argue that community empowerment is so much more than passing over decision-making power, especially if people within said community settings do not have genuine options due to their marginalisation. They may also lack the capacity to make autonomous choices. This applies to those within communities, as well as to whole communities. Second, if health promoters enhance community control, they may find themselves advocating, funding and supporting interventions that they see as problematic. Third, resource limitations also result in ethical challenges when using bottom-up approaches, because priorities have to be determined, and these may be influenced by more powerful community groups. Community empowerment as a health promotion goal is also questionable, as it can only be a means rather than an end in itself.

lead to different ethical debates, and questions. Table 3.2 outlines some illustrative political and associated ethical positions.

As Table 3.2 shows, different political viewpoints result in ethical debates, so in light of this, have you considered where your own ideological position in relation to structure and agency, and what this means for your ethical standpoint? Please take some time to carry out Reflection on Practice 3.2.

Reflection on ethics and values, is indeed complex, and therefore when interventions are used in health promotion contexts, criticisms arise. For example, programmes focusing on individuals and their lifestyles

Table 3.2 Political and ethical positions associated with health promotion interventions

Political position	Level of intervention	Ethical stance
Conservative	Low or no intervention – individuals need to take responsibility for themselves.	The state does not have a right to intrude into people's personal life (Kelly and Charlton, 1995; Fitzpatrick, 2001). However, critics argue that ethically this stance may reinforce stigma and contribute towards 'deviance amplification', labelling or moral condemnation (Nettleton and Bunton, 1995; Lowenberg, 1995; Smith, 2000; Cross et al., 2020), for those not taking responsibility.
New Right	Neo-liberal approaches are also focused on low levels of intervention, in which individuals need to take responsibility for themselves, though they can be nudged.	Lifestyle choices are decisions which individuals make, not governments, so individuals should have autonomy and the right to choose their own health behaviours (Minkler, 1999; Jochelson, 2006). However, if nudges are used to 'encourage' choices, many ethical questions are raised (see Box 3.2).
New Left	This political stance accounts for wider processes influencing health outcomes. People are seen as needing support to build competencies to challenge wider determinants, through participation.	Individualising health issues does not account for the complex social factors which underpin behavioural choice and ignores the broader context in which personal behaviours are embedded (Green and Raeburn, 1988; Laverack, 2004; Staten et al., 2005., Marmot, 2017). Ignoring this blames people for their poor health (Nettleton and Bunton, 1995; Cross et al., 2020).
Marxist, Socialist	Class and economic position are seen as fundamentally important in predicting life chances. Therefore, redistribution is required. In addition, commercial interests are understood as influencing health.	Ethically, power needs to be shared more widely. Commercial interests need to be tackled to improve health. Lee and Crosbie (2020) highlight the role of unethical commercial interests underpinning health problems linked to tobacco use, alcohol consumption and unhealthy diet.

(Continued)

Table 3.2 (Continued)

Political position	Level of intervention	Ethical stance
Ecological	This position acknowledges the complex array of factors that affect health, and so incorporates both left and right ideological perspectives. In such approaches attention is focused on both individuals and structures.	Ethically such models of health promotion practice, attempt to unite the goals of enabling people to control and improve their own health with larger structural objective to create healthier conditions for people to live in (Porter, 2016).

Reflection on Practice 3.2: Ideology and ethics in relation to structure and agency

Revisit Table 3.2, and think about where you would place yourself in terms of your political views. Thinking about your own ideological and political views or the political perspectives of the government in the country you live in debate the following interventions:

1 Laws to safeguard people such as compulsory seatbelt wearing. Should people then have full agency to decide whether they should or should not use seatbelts, and what about the ethics of this approach in relation to children's decision-making, as well as other individuals who are deemed to lack capacity?

2 State intervention, especially in relation to health improvement for those living in the most vulnerable conditions, for example food vouchers to support healthy eating, regeneration of neighbourhoods, specific service support as per area needs? Ethically in terms of health promotion practice, do state actors always know what is best for all communities?

are criticised for failing to tackle macro-level environmental conditions (Kelly and Charlton, 1995; Nettleton and Bunton, 1995; Cross et al., 2020) despite such work existing in a political context in the global north where many governments do not intervene at such a policy level (Warwick-Booth, 2022). However, where governments do intervene they are often subjected to criticisms of them operating as a nanny state (Lupton, 1995). Commercial interests are also at play, working to challenge policy measures for example around healthy diets by calling governments paternalistic and using the label of nanny state in a nefarious unethical manner to serve their own interests (Steele et al., 2021). In presenting different positions in Table 3.2, it is important to note that there is nothing inherently 'good' or 'bad' in approaching health promotion from an individualist or collectivist position (Breslow, 1990); but complexity has to be acknowledged, to avoid problematic consequences (Davison and Davey Smith, 1995; Minkler, 1999; Rutten and Gelius, 2011). Rutten and Gelius (2011) clearly demonstrate the need for health promotion approaches that account for the interplay of both structure and agency. They use a case study from Germany, to show how the interaction between structure and agency at a multi-model level, led to the establishment of a women-only time at a local swimming pool, increasing the physical activity levels of this target group.

Finally, Gregg and O'Hara's (2007) discussion of the values and principles for health promotion in a complex world, need consideration in relation to ethics. They highlight several challenges which still need consideration in relation to the ethics of health promotion practice based upon their review of literature from which they listed holistic, ecological and salutogenic models of ethical health promotion practice, comparing and contrasting these to more traditional approaches. As Chapter 2 outlined earlier, there are several ethical frameworks available to those working in health promotion. They argue that contemporary models of health promotion are underpinned by organic values, focus on health as a resource for living, and are determined by equity as well as underpinned by participatory empowering practices. Therefore, these can be argued to be more ethical approaches. In comparison, traditional models of health promotion practice are linked to less ethical values as they were more reductionist, more biomedical in focus, patriarchal, and likely to limit autonomy. In identifying these complexities, Gregg and O'Hara (2007, p. 7) argue that '*a system of values and principles would assist practitioners to respond to complex health issues that have multiple interrelated determinants*' because challenges remain in using values to inform practice (see Box 3.3).

Summary

This chapter has highlighted some of the key ethical debates in health promotion, exploring these through discussing moral injustices arising from interventions, as well as the ethics of empowerment approaches. Issues such as rights and responsibilities, agency and structure, the role of the state in health promotion, and the potential limits of autonomy were

---

Box 3.3   Gregg and O'Hara's (2007) challenges for health promotion practice

1 Lack of agreement on the core values and principles of health promotion: there are several lists of principles and some commonalities when comparing these; however, there is no single recognised set of principles applicable to all health promotion activity.
2 Working with the values and principles of health promotion: there is also an issue for any practitioner wishing to apply values in their practice, because specific guidance on doing this is lacking. Well-used health promotion models discussed in the literature are technically focused, rather than discussing the values underpinning actions associated with them.
3 Using the values and principles in practice: there are many interpretations of values which makes using them difficult in practice. Participation and empowerment for example, are described as strategies, ways of working and as outcomes.
4 The gap between modern and conventional health promotion values and principles: some contemporary health promotion work remains aligned to more traditional, biomedical approaches, linked to funding which focuses practice on physical ill-health rather than more holistic contemporary ideals such as wellbeing.

---

all considered. The chapter used the Nuffield Ladder of Intervention to highlight key ethical questions about interventions, personal choice, and balancing the greater good against personal freedom. An in-depth exploration of Nudge Theory and Choice Architecture, plus the concepts of structure and agency also raised a number of ethical issues. Finally Gregg and O'Hara's (2007) values and principles were also considered in relation to the ethics of contemporary health promotion practice.

Key points

• Tensions are found within these key ethical debates, when attention is paid to the ethics of interventions compared to the rights of people to choose their own health practices.
• There are many ongoing ethical debates taking place in health promotion, linked to political viewpoints, and associated ways of working. The complexity of structural determinants and individual agency in social contexts, contribute to these ethical debates.

- It remains important for practitioners to understand and explore ethical debates in the discipline of health promotion, through comparing values and principles that underpin practice.

Further reading

Gardner, J. and Biko, S. (2014) Ethical issues in health promotion *South African Journal of Bioethics and Law*, 7, (1), 30–33.
This short article discusses many of the key questions raised in this chapter, around the ethical issues relating to practices which intend to support people to achieve better health. The authors debate efficacy as well as autonomy in relation to behaviour change.
Nuffield Bioethics Council (2007) *Public health: ethical issues*. Retrieved from https://www.nuffieldbioethics.org/publications/public-health
This is a detailed report outlining the ladder of intervention, and accompanying debates about costs, benefits, liberty, and the role of state, media, industry and other parties. The report concludes that the state and other organisations are obligated to society, and therefore justifies state intervention in health promotion.
Tengland, P. (2016) Behaviour change or empowerment: On the ethics of health-promotion goals *Health Care Anal*, 24, 24–46.
This article debates the goals of practice, attempting to clarify these, and evaluate the strengths and weaknesses of behaviour change approaches, compared to empowerment work. The author highlights moral and ethical problems with both approaches.

References

Action on Salt (2023) *Call to reduce salt content in bread as three in four products are as salty as a packet of crisps in just one slice*. Retrieved from https://www.actiononsalt.org.uk/salt-surveys/2023/bread/
Ananthapavan, J., Peterson, A. and Sacks, G. (2018) Paying people to lose weight: The effectiveness of financial incentives provided by health insurers for the prevention and management of overweight and obesity – A systematic review. *Obesity Reviews*, 19, 605–613.
Arno, A. and Thomas, S. (2016) The efficacy of nudge theory strategies in influencing adult dietary behaviour: A systematic review and meta-analysis. *BMC Public Health*, 16 (1), 1–11.
Bakhshi, F., Shojaeizadeh, D., Sadeghi, R., Taghdisi, M.H. and Nedjat, S. (2017) The relationship between individual empowerment and health-promoting lifestyle among women NGOs in northern Iran. *Electron Physician*, 9 (2), 3690–3698.
Barton, H. and Grant, M. (2006) A health map for the local human habitat. *The Journal for the Royal Society for the Promotion of Health*, 126 (6), 252–253.
Baum, F. (2003) *The New Public Health*. Melbourne, Oxford University Press.
Bourdieu, P. (1984) *Distinction. A Social Critique of the Judgement of Taste*. London, Routledge.

Braithwaite, R.S. (2022) Are healthful behavior change policies ever unethical? *Journal of Public Health Policy*, 43, 685–695.

Braunack-Mayer, A. and Louise, J. (2008) The ethics of community empowerment: Tensions in health promotion theory and practice. *Promotion & Education*, 15 (3), 5–8.

Breslow, L. (1990) A health promotion primer for the 1990s. *Health Affairs*, 9, 6–21.

Brown, R.C., Maslen, H. and Savulescu, H. (2019) Against moral responsibilisation of health: Prudential responsibility and health promotion. *Public Health Ethics*, 12 (2), 114–129.

Cavico, F.J. and Mujtaba, B.G. (2013) Health and wellness policy ethics. *International Journal of Health Policy and Management*, 1 (2), 111–113.

Cho, H.L., Grady, C., Tarzian, A., Povar, G., Mangal, J. and Danis, M. (2020) Patient and family descriptions of ethical concerns. *American Journal of Bioethics*, 20 (6), 52–64.

Cheung, D and Ip, E. C. (2020) COVID-19 lockdowns: A public mental health ethics perspective. *Asian Bioethics Review*, 12 (4), 503–510.

Chriss, J.J. (2015) Nudging and social marketing. *Social Science and Public Policy*, 52, 54–61.

Cockerham, W.C., Rutten, A. and Abel, T. (1997) Conceptualising contemporary health lifestyles: Moving beyond Weber. *The Sociological Quarterly*, 38 (2), 321–342.

Cockerham, W.C. (2007) *Social Causes of Health and Disease*. Cambridge, Polity Press.

Cross, R., Davis, S. and O'Neil, I. (2017) *Health Communication: Theoretical and Critical Perspectives*. Cambridge, Polity Press.

Cross, R.M., Warwick-Booth, L., Rowlands, S., Woodall, J., O'Neil, I. and Foster, S. (2020) *Health Promotion. Global Principals and Practice*. 2nd Edn. Wallingford, CABI.

Cross, R., Woodall, J. and Warwick-Booth, L. (2017) Empowerment: Challenges in measurement? *Global Health Promotion*, 26 (2), 93–96.

Dahlgren, G. and Whitehead, M. (1991) *Policies and Strategies to Promote Social Equity in Health*. Stockholm, Institute for Futures Studies.

Davison, C. and Davey Smith, G. (1995) The baby and the bath water: Examining socio-cultural and free-market critiques of health promotion. In: Bunton, R., Nettleton, S. and Burrows (Eds.), *The Sociology of Health Promotion*. London, Routledge.

Department of Health and Social Care (2022) *Restricting promotions of products high in fat, sugar or salt by location and by volume price: Implementation guidance*. Retrieved from https://www.gov.uk/government/publications/restricting-promotions-of-products-high-in-fat-sugar-or-salt-by-location-and-by-volume-price/restricting-promotions-of-products-high-in-fat-sugar-or-salt-by-location-and-by-volume-price-implementation-guidance

Downie, R.S., Tannahill, C. and Tannahill, A. (1996) *Health Promotion. Models and Values*. Oxford, Oxford University Press.

Ensaff, H. (2021) A nudge in The right direction: The role of food choice architecture in changing populations diet. *Proceedings of the Nutrition Society*, 80, 195–206.

Fitzpatrick, M. (2001) *The Tyranny of Health*. London, Routledge.
Frith, L. (2020) Lockdown, public good and equality during COVID-19. *Journal of Medical Ethics*, 46, 713–714.
Gagliani, M. (2019) *Smoking ban in the United Kingdom*. Retrieved from https://www.centreforpublicimpact.org/case-study/smoking-ban-united-kingdom/
Gardner, J. and Biko, S. (2014) Ethical issues in health promotion. *South African Journal of Bioethics and Law*, 7 (1), 30–33.
Giddens, A. (1984) *The Constitution of Society. Outline of the Theory of Structuration*. Cambridge, Polity Press.
Goiana-da-Silva, F., Cruz-E-Silva, D., Bartlett, O., Vasconcelos, J., Morais Nunes, A., Ashrafian, H., Miraldo, M., Machado, M.D.C., Araújo, F. and Darzi, A. (2020) The ethics of taxing sugar-sweetened beverages to improve public health. *Frontiers in Public Health*, 16 (8), 110. http://dx.doi.org/10.3389/fpubh.2020.00110
Gray, S. (2013) How far up the ladder should we go? *Journal of Public Health*, 35 (3), 353.
Green, J. (2004) The power to choose. *Promotion & Education*, 11, 2–3.
Green, L.W. and Raeburn, J.M. (1988) Health promotion. What is it? What will it become? *Health Promotion*, 3, 151–159.
Gregg, J. and O'Hara, L. (2007) Values and principles evident in current health promotion practice. *Health Promotion Journal of Australia*, 18 (1), 7–11.
Griffiths, P.E. and West, C. (2015) A balanced intervention ladder: Promoting autonomy through public health action *Public Health*, 1092–1098.
Guttman, N. (2017) Ethical issues in health promotion and communication interventions. *Oxford Research Encyclopedia of Communication*. Retrieved from https://oxfordre.com/communication/view/10.1093/a
Halpern, S.D., Madison, K.M. and Volpp, K.G. (2009) Patients as mercenaries?: The ethics of using financial incentives in the war on unhealthy behaviors. *Circ Cardiovasc Qual Outcomes*, 2 (5), 514–516.
Hastings, G. and Stead, M. (2006) Social marketing. In: MacDowall, W., Bonell, C. and Davies, M. (Eds.), *Health Promotion Practice*. Open University Press, Maidenhead, pp. 139–151.
Huitink, M., Poelman, M.P., van den Eynde, E., Jacob, C., Seidell, J.C. and Coosje Dijkstra, S. (2020) Social norm nudges in shopping trolleys to promote vegetable purchases: A quasi-experimental study in a supermarket in a deprived urban area in the Netherlands *Appetite*, 151, 104655. https://doi.org/10.1016/j.appet.2020.104655
Jochelson, K. (2006) Nanny or steward? The role of government in public health. *Public Health*, 120, 1149–1155.
Kelly, M.P. and Charlton, B. (1995) The modern and postmodern in health promotion. In: Bunton, R., Nettleton, R. and Burrows (Eds.), *The Sociology of Health Promotion*. London, Routledge.
Kickbusch, I. (1986) Issues in health promotion. *Health Promotion*, 1, 437–442.
Kwoh, L. (2013) Shape up or pay up: Firms put in new health penalties. *The Wall Street Journal*, 6-7, A1–10.
Larsen, E.L. and Manderson, L. (2009) "A good spot": Health promotion discourse, Healthy cities and heterogeneity in contemporary Denmark. *Health & Place*, 15, 606–613.

Laverack, G. (2004) *Health Promotion Practice: Power and Empowerment.* London, Sage.

Ledderer, L., Kjaer, M., Madsen, E.K., Busch, J. and Fage-Butler, A. (2020) Nudging in public health lifestyle interventions: A systematic literature review and metasynthesis. *Health Education and Behaviour,* 47 (5), 749–764.

Lee, K. and Crosbie, E. (2020) Understanding structure and agency as commercial determinants of health. *International Journal Health Policy Management,* 9 (7), 315–318.

Linhorst, D.M., Hamilton, G., Young, E. and Eckert, A. (2002) Opportunities and barriers to empowering people with severe mental illness through participation in treatment planning. *Social Work,* 47, 425–434.

Lin, Y., Osman, M. and Ashcroft, R. (2017) Nudge: Concept, effectiveness, and ethics. *Basic and Applied Social Psychology,* 39 (6), 293–306.

Lodge, M. and Wegrich, K. (2016) The rationality paradox of nudge: Rational tools of government in a world of bounded rationality. *Law & Policy,* 38 (3), 250–267.

Loibl, C., Sunstein, C.R., Rauber, J. and Reisch, L.A. (2018) Which Europeans like nudges? Approval and controversy in four European countries. *The Journal of Consumer Affairs,* 3, 655–688.

Lowenberg, J.S. (1995) Health promotion and the "ideology of choice". *Public Health Nursing,* 12, 319–323.

Lupton, D. (1995) *The Imperative of Health. Public Health and the Regulated Body.* London, Sage.

Marmot, M. (2017) The health gap: The challenge of an unequal world: The argument *International Journal of Epidemiology,* 46, 1312–1318.

Marteau, T.M., Ogilvie, D., Roland, M. and Suhrcke, M. (2011) Judging nudging: Can nudging improve population health? *British Medical Journal,* 342, 263–265.

Milio, N. (1986) *Promoting Health Through Public Policy.* Ottawa, Canadian Public Health Association.

Mills, C.M. (2023) Ethics of recommending weight loss in older adults: A case study. *Clinical Ethics,* 18 (1), 120–127.

Minkler, M. (1999) Personal responsibility for health? A review of the arguments and the evidence at century's end. *Health Education & Behavior,* 26, 121–140.

Naidoo, J. and Wills, J. (2009) *Foundations for Health Promotion.* London & Amsterdam, Elsevier Health Sciences.

Nettleton, S. (1995) *The Sociology of Health and Illness.* Bristol, Polity Press.

Nettleton, S. and Bunton, R. (1995) Sociological critiques of health promotion. In: Bunton, R., Nettleton, S. and Burrows, R. (Eds.), *The Sociology of Health Promotion.* London, Routledge.

Nuffield Bioethics Council (2007) *Public health: Ethical issues.* Retrieved from https://www.nuffieldbioethics.org/publications/public-health

Porter, C.M. (2016) Revisiting Precede–Proceed: A leading model for ecological and ethical health promotion. *Health Education Journal,* 75 (6), 753–764.

Rissel, C. (1994) Empowerment: The holy grail of health promotion? *Health Promotion International,* 9, 39–47.

Robinson, E. (2020) *Nudge acceptance in developing countries: Ethical (or unnecessary) litmus test?* Retrieved from https://bppblog.com/2020/09/08/nudge-acceptance-in-developing-countries-ethical-or-unnecessary-litmus-test/

Rodwell, C.M. (1996) An analysis of the concept of empowerment. *Journal of Advanced Nursing*, 23, 305–313.

Rouyard, T., Engelen, B., Papanikitas, A. and Nakamura, R. (2022) Boosting healthier choices. *BMJ*, 376, e064225. http://dx.doi.org/10.1136/bmj-2021-064225

Rutten, A. and Gelius, P. (2011) The interplay of structure and agency in health promotion: Integrating a concept of structural change and the policy dimension into a multi-level model and applying it to health promotion principles and practice. *Social Science and Medicine*, 73, 953–959.

Schwartz, B. and Cheek, N.N. (2017) Choice, freedom and well-being: Considerations for public policy. *Behavioural Public Policy*, 1 (1), 106–121.

Selinger, E. and Whyte, K. (2011) Is there a right way to nudge? The practice and ethics of choice architecture. *Sociology Compass*, 5/10, 923–935.

Sibeon, R. (1999) Agency, structure, and social chance as cross-disciplinary concepts. *Politics*, 19, 139–144.

Smith, C. (2000) Healthy prisons: A contradiction in terms? *The Howard Journal of Criminal Justice*, 39, 339–353.

Spencer, G. (2015) 'Troubling' moments in health promotion: Unpacking the ethics of empowerment. *Health Promotion Journal of Australia*, 26, 205–209.

Staten, R., Miller, K., Noland, M.P. and Rayens, M.K. (2005) College students' physical activity: Application of an ecological perspective. *American Journal of Health Studies*, 20, 58–65.

Steele, M., Mialon, M., Browne, S., Campbell, N. and Finucane, F. (2021) Obesity, public health ethics and the nanny state. *Ethics, Medicine and Public Health*, 19, 100724. http://dx.doi.org/10.1016/j.jemep.2021.100724

Tengland, P. (2016) Behaviour change or empowerment: On the ethics of health-promotion goals. *Health Care Anal*, 24, 24–46.

Thaler, R.H. and Sunstein, C.R. (2009) *Nudge: Improving Decisions About Health, Wealth and Happiness*. New International Edition. London, Penguin.

Thompson, N. (2007) *Power and Empowerment*. Lyme Regis, Russell House Publishing.

Tones, K. (1998) Health promotion: Empowering choice. In: Myers, L.B. and Midence, K. (Eds.), *Adherence to Treatment in Medical Conditions*. Amsterdam, Harwood Academic Publishers.

Tones, K. and Tilford, S. (2001) *Health Promotion. Effectiveness, Efficiency and Equity*. Cheltenham, Nelson Thornes.

Ujewe, S.J. (2018) Moral residue and health justice for the global south: Addressing past issues through current interventions and research. *Developing World Bioethics*, 20 (2), 96–104.

van der Eijk, Y. and Porter, G. (2013) Human rights and ethical considerations for a tobacco-free generation. *Tobacco Control*, 24, 238–242.

Wallerstein, N. (1992) Powerlessness, empowerment, and health: Implications for health promotion programs. *American Journal of Health Promotion*, 6, 197–205.

Ward, D. and Mullender, A. (1991) Empowerment and oppression: An indissoluble pairing for contemporary social work. *Critical Social Policy*, 11, 21–29.

Warwick-Booth, L. (2022) *Social Inequality*. 3rd Edn. London, Sage.

Warwick-Booth, L., Cross, R. and Lowcock, D. (2021) *Contemporary Health Studies: An Introduction*. 2nd Edn. Cambridge, Polity.

Woodall, J., Warwick-Booth, L. and Cross, R. (2012) Has empowerment lost its power? *Health Education Research*, 27 (4), 742–745.

World Health Organization (WHO) (2017) *Taxes on Sugary Drinks: Why Do It?* Geneva, World Health Organization.

World Health Organization (WHO) (2022) *New WHO signature initiative shows raising alcohol taxes could save 130 000 lives per year.* Retrieved from https://www.who.int/europe/news/item/23-02-2022-new-who-signature-initiative-shows-raising-alcohol-taxes-could-save-130-000-lives-per-year

World Health Organization (WHO) (2023) *Salt reduction.* Retrieved from https://www.who.int/news-room/fact-sheets/detail/salt-reduction

4 Ethics in health promotion practice

Introduction

This chapter explores some of the main ethical considerations, tensions and challenges in health promotion practice. Within in the chapter the fundamental question of whether aspects of health promotion practice are indeed unethical and may even contradict the key aim of improving health and reducing inequalities and social injustices, will be discussed. The chapter considers a range of questions and will conclude with a discussion on whether an ethical code of practice, frequently discussed by some, is necessary in order to provide an ethical framework for health promotion practice.

By the end of this chapter the reader should be able to:

- Understand the ethical tensions in health promotion practice;
- Gain insight into how some, well-meaning, health promotion interventions can have adverse impacts and may be unethical;
- Consider whether a code of ethics is necessary for health promoters to inform their practice.

The exaggerated claims of health promotion?

Fundamental to the issue of the ethics of health promotion practice is whether health promotion itself is an ethical discipline – based on a sound knowledge base – that indeed achieves improved health for individuals and communities. Guttman (2017) summarises this in two key questions: first, does it (health promotion) promote people's health and second, whom does it actually benefit?

Ever since the foundational pillars of health promotion were discussed and consolidated in the Ottawa Charter (WHO, 1986), individuals have suggested that the field is 'riddled' with ethical problems (Williams, 1985) and many have suggested that health promotion practitioners and academics need to take ethics more seriously (Hubley et al.,

DOI: 10.4324/9781003308317-4

2021). Several commentators though have continued to point out that health promotion has serious ethical flaws in its conceptualisation and practice. James Le Fanu's (1994) book, written during the time when health promotion was seen as a key mechanism to achieving good population health and well supported by international and national agencies, was one of the first to be highly sceptical of health promotion practice. He, and other contributors to the book, questioned the ethics of health promotion directly and claimed that much of the enthusiasm for health promotion was based on exaggerated claims, underpinned by an indifferent and relatively weak evidence base. Health promotion has strived to legitimise itself against more medical approaches to prevention through gathering better evidence of what works, but there has sometimes been resentment towards health promotion interventions by medical professions due to the discipline not perceived to have a robust evidence base (perhaps underpinned by sound-randomised controlled trials) and this has led to some questioning the ethical basis for resourcing health promotion programmes and interventions (South and Tilford, 2000; Green et al., 2019). The adage that prevention is better and cheaper than cure is, therefore, contested (see Case Study 4.1 as an example).

Case Study 4.1 Ethics and exclusion: an example from Sure Start, UK

Sure Start is a UK Government initiative that seeks to reduce and alleviate child poverty and improve health outcomes in children under four years and their families who live in socially deprived communities in England. Sure Start does not have a prescribed model or intervention, but it does include: outreach or home visiting; family support; support for good quality play, learning, and childcare experiences; primary and community healthcare; advice about child and family health and development; and support for people with special needs, including help in accessing specialised services. Community participation is central to the mission of these programmes (Belsky et al., 2006).

Despite the promise of Sure Start, evidence has shown that the effects are minimal with some indication of adverse effects in the most disadvantaged families (with respect to mothers who were teenagers when the child was born, lone parents and workless households) (Rutter, 2006). Socially deprived families with better access to personal resources may have been better able to take advantage of Sure Start, which may have left those with fewer personal resources (such as young mothers and lone parents) with less access to services. Evidence also showed that more socially deprived parents may perceive the extra attention of service providers in Sure Starts stressful and intrusive (Belsky et al., 2006).

So, how can a well-meaning health promotion intervention cause more harm than good for some families in some contexts? (See Reflection on Practice 4.1 to consider this more widely.) Sure Start is a universal area-based intervention for all families with children living in a designated area. This brings many positives as it is open to all and does not make people feel stigmatised for attending. Sure Start focussed on communities with high levels of deprivation, but according to Rutter (2006), this had two consequences: it meant that there would be considerable individual variation in the degree of disadvantage experienced by individual families (because most areas in the UK are fairly heterogeneous in nature), and it meant that many seriously disadvantaged families would be excluded because the area in which they lived was not so disadvantaged overall (because many disadvantaged families do not live in disadvantaged areas). Other critics have argued that Sure Start is overly individualist focussing on the manifestations of deprivation rather than the root causes of structural inequality (see section on the ethics of lifestyle pre-occupation later in the chapter). Its focus was too readily on the manipulation of the child's immediate environment, primarily individual maternal behaviour, rather than challenging broader societal issues (Clarke, 2006).

Reflection on Practice 4.1

Try to consider in more detail who you feel are the beneficiaries of health promotion interventions and who perhaps 'miss out' on any benefits and why. Why might certain groups be excluded from seemingly well-meaning programmes and consider how this can exacerbate, rather than reduce, health inequalities.

Returning to Guttman's (2017) question as to who benefits from health promotion, the notion that health promotion endeavours could increase, rather than narrow, health inequalities is a moot point. However, there is convincing evidence that suggests that efforts of health promoters to make things 'fairer' has resulted in making things far worse. Thereby reinforcing the view that health promotion efforts are over-inflated and potentially unethical. The settings approach to health promotion, as an example, is a cornerstone of health promotion practice (Woodall and Cross, 2021). Whilst the original policy references to settings typically concerned environments such as cities, schools, workplaces and hospitals (Barić, 1992; Department of Health, 1992), this was a narrow view of a setting. Consequently, early settings based approaches only managed to focus on 'legitimate sites of practice' (Green et al., 2000, p. 25) by focussing on large-scale, identifiable and easily accessible organisations. This potentially exacerbated health inequalities (Speller, 2006; Dooris and Hunter, 2007) by failing to consider groups who are found outside of these formal organisations (e.g. the unemployed, illegal immigrants, children who truant from school and the homeless).

Health promotion is often tacitly viewed as a 'good thing' with laudable intentions to benefit individuals and communities. Indeed, it is naively presumed that health promotion is a risk-free pursuit, which, at worst, may do no good (Skrabanek, 1990). That said, there are legitimate claims that health promotion has significant side-effects that recipients of interventions and programmes may be unaware.

Health promotion practice and its unethical side-effects?

Health promotion, as frequently conceptualised and practiced, has a morality dimension in-built within its fabric (Green et al., 2019) (the link between ethics and morals were discussed in Chapter 2). This is especially the case for those subscribing to more individualised notions of health promotion where education and attempts to shift behaviour are the cornerstone of practice (health promotion does, of course, have a whole spectrum of intervention approaches, see Beattie (1991) as an example, and whilst the focus here is on behaviour change and individualised strategies, Chapter 3 discusses the ethical challenges associated with policy approaches which tackles structural issues). In many cases, behavioural choices become the focus of health education and are frequently delineated into being 'healthy' (good) and 'unhealthy' (bad) and this is seen largely in the discourse surrounding diet, physical activity, smoking and alcohol consumption:

> *Public health messages specifying the 'right' kind of lifestyle are pervasive, instructing us to (at last count) consume five portions of fruit and vegetables a day, engage in 150 min of moderate physical activity per week, refrain from smoking entirely and drink no more than 14 units of alcohol per week.*
>
> (Brown, 2018, p. 1005)

Individuals and communities opting to pursue 'unhealthy' choices are often condemned for such decisions. Health promoters are often seen as the moral arbiters and the professional group setting the categorisation of whether a behaviour is 'good' or 'bad'. Indeed the word 'promotion' is in itself about convincing other people that they need, or ought to have, what the promoter wants them to have (Williams, 1985). Such conceptualisations that health promotion concerns 'marketing' and 'selling' rather than 'enhancement' and 'empowerment' (Catford, 2004), is far from the original principles of health promotion when first envisaged. However, such a discourse of 'promoting' what is right, places specific (frequently middle-class) health values on a pedestal to be attained (Nettleton, 1995), rather than recognising that health means very different things to different people (Scriven, 2017). This is observed most acutely when lower socio-economic groups do not conform to the morality decided by health promoters and are:

> ... *typically portrayed as those who fail to take up the exhortations of health promoters, who deliberately expose themselves to health risks rather than 'rationally' avoiding them, and who, therefore, require greater surveillance and regulation.*
>
> (Smith, 2000, p. 344)

Some argue that health promoters often do believe that a healthy life is one where people prioritise health rather than hedonism or seeming recklessness (Woodall and Rowlands, 2020) and commentators have historically criticised the morality inherent in health promotion discourse. Health promoters instinctively try to create 'better' social systems through health improvement and some have suggested that health promotion aims to create a 'good' society. For many health promoters then, optimum health is 'good' but there are other 'good' things in life too that may complement or indeed inhibit optimum health (Carter et al., 2012). This brings health and morality back to the forefront. Fitzgerald (1994) comparing smoking and skiing argued how both pursuits could lead to injury, may be costly and are clearly risky but that one is regarded as being more socially acceptable than the other. Whilst perhaps designed to be purposely provocative and flippant, it indeed highlights the challenge and contradiction of a moral perspective in health promotion. Where does this leave the health promoter though? Is simply suggesting unfettered freedom and rights to make decisions about their health the most suitable course of action, however 'foolish' such choices may be? We will consider this further later in the chapter.

Analysis demonstrates that the ability to make autonomous and free choices in relation to our health is flawed, or at least majorly constrained and so suggesting that this is not the case is unethical. Socio-economic and educational factors, just as two examples, consistently show how choices are influenced (Green et al., 2019). It is therefore a continued tension to see health promotion approaches and campaigns continuing to adopt a lifestyle focus with strong moral undertones when much of the evidence suggests that people's lifestyle decisions are manifestations of the socio-environmental conditions. This was highlighted very recently by the COVID-19 pandemic (see Case Study 4.2).

The side-effect of a moral dimension in health promotion practice is stigmatisation and marginalisation for those opting not to conform with the direction or advice of health promoters. Put simply, it is an unethical

---

Case Study 4.2   The pitfalls of personalisation rhetoric in time of health crisis: COVID-19 pandemic and cracks on neoliberal ideologies

Abstract

The rise of the COVID-19 pandemic has exposed the incongruity of individualisation ideologies that position individuals at the centre of health care, by contributing, making informed decisions and exercising choice regarding their health options and lifestyle considerations. When confronted with a global health threat, government across the world, have understood that the rhetoric of individualisation, personal responsibility and personal choice would only led to disastrous national health consequences. In other words, individual choice offers a poor criterion to guide the health and wellbeing of a population. This reality has forced many advanced economies around the world to suspend their pledges to 'small government', individual responsibility and individual freedom, opting instead for a more rebalanced approach to economic and health outcomes with an increasing role for institutions and mutualisation. For many marginalised communities, individualisation ideologies and personalisation approaches have never worked. On the contrary, they have exacerbated social and health inequalities by benefiting affluent individuals who possess the educational, cultural and economic resources required to exercise 'responsibility', avert risks and adopt health protecting behaviours. The individualisation of the management of risk has also further stigmatised the poor by shifting the blame for poor health outcomes from government to individuals.

Source: Cardona (2020, p. 714)

side-effect of seemingly well-meaning practice. Indeed, Becker warned that health promotion was a 'new religion' where illness was a punishment for those who chose 'unhealthy' ways (Becker, 1986). Crawford (1980) suggested that the ideology of blaming the victim here underplayed what he termed, the 'assault' on health caused by structural and environmental forces. This stigmatisation is probably the most widely discussed unintended effect of health promotion interventions in the literature (Gugglberger, 2018). A whole plethora of conditions can be stigmatised as a result of moral framing in health promotion (Brown, 2018). This is amplified through the negative stereotyping of those with behavioural risk factors in the media, such as individuals being overweight or choosing to smoke (Brown et al., 2019). Whilst the role of individual choice plays some role, alcohol, saturated fat, salt, nicotine, etc., are powerfully addictive and heavily promoted by commercial interest (Beauchamp, 1987). Victim-blaming is common and more recently, there are concerning examples of victim-blaming becoming more prevalent in the media and in public discourse, especially in relation to sexual assault victims – examples of victim blaming may be asking someone why they dressed a certain way or if they consumed alcohol prior to the assault (Wilson et al., 2022). The impact of stigmatisation can be profound and is contradictory to the tenets of health promotion and yet poorly conceived programmes can exacerbate, rather than alleviate, poor health outcomes.

The ethics of health communication

Health communication is a common strategy used to influence behaviour change or to raise awareness of particular issues, it can take a myriad of forms (online, visual, written, oral) and can cover a plethora of issues (Cross et al., 2017). One approach within health communication strategy is to incite 'fear', 'guilt' and 'anxiety' (see Reflection on Practice 4.2) in the recipient and to trigger an emotional response which may contribute to addressing health behaviours or in raising consciousness of an issue. It is a health communication technique that seeks to provide, for example, images or text that shock people or raise an emotional response (for instance on the dangers of substance use or the dangers of obesity) which will then be resolved by individuals changing their behaviour or thinking differently. Originally theorists suggested that mild fear could arouse interest, create concern and lead to change, but that too much fear can lead to people denying and rejecting the message (Hubley et al., 2021). Getting the level of 'fear' correct though is difficult and indeed subject – what causes an emotional response for one person may not in another (Demirtaş-Madran, 2021). That said, recent analysis has shown how fear can be harnessed effectively to support health promoting

Reflection on Practice 4.2

What fear appeals do you recall seeing and what impact did they have on you? Was there a situation where the message resonated and made you feel differently about yourself or others?

Recent research during the COVID-19 pandemic used the following message to explore fear and arousal response (Heffner et al., 2021).

The coronavirus is coming for you. When it does, your health-care system will be overwhelmed. Your fellow citizens will be turned away at the hospital doors. Exhausted healthcare workers will break down. Millions will die. The only way to prevent this crisis is social distancing today.

How would you react to such messaging? How does it make you feel? Do you feel you would react in a positive or negative way to this?

In what situations do you think using fear is a well-founded approach to raising awareness of an issue or in encouraging behaviour modification. Under what circumstances could this be seen as an ethical and effective approach?

actions. As an illustration, fear was the main predictor of positive behaviour changes associated with the prevention of spreading COVID-19 (Demirtaş-Madran, 2021).

Harm minimisation communication has also been identified as an ethical problem for health promotion. As an example, *When the Fun Stops, Stop*, is a prominent 'responsible gambling' campaign in the UK which was overseen by the Senet Group – a group initiated and funded by the gambling industry (van Schalkwyk et al., 2021). This message is widely deployed, but has been criticised for its suggestion that gambling is fun and that individuals are responsible for keeping it that way (Rintoul, 2022). Indeed the evidence showed that *When the Fun Stops, Stop* had no protective effect as a safer gambling message (Newall et al., 2022). Similar evidence is seen in the alcohol sector where harm minimisation messages and health communication (funded by the alcohol industry) have the potential to make behaviour change far more difficult (Petticrew et al., 2020). This raises two important issues for health promotion practice – first, how powerful health communication techniques can be and how they can manipulate behaviours;

messages that seem well intended can have a more powerful effect and 'nudge' people into acting in ways that might not be expected (Chapter 3 has provided a more detailed analysis on this). Second, the importance of research and evaluation in testing health communication techniques to ensure that the validity of the health communication message and minimising unintended consequences (Chapter 6 has more on this).

The ethics of lifestyle interventions in health promotion

Advocates, scholars and practitioners of health promotion have recognised that the social determinants of health, outlined by a range of scholars including Marmot and colleagues (Marmot, 1996, 2002, 2010; Marmot et al., 2008, 2020a, 2020b), are central in tackling health inequalities in society. These social determinants are the factors that drive good health and preclude some groups from achieving their fullest health potential. Nonetheless, policy effects in addressing broader social, economic and environmental influences on health have been modest and inequalities still remain (Williams and Fullagar, 2019). Behavioural approaches are instead frequently used by health promoters in promoting healthy lifestyles and remain the raison d'être of the health promotion practitioner, despite dubious evidence of long-term effectiveness (Woodall and Rowlands, 2020).

There is an ethical implication of health promotion practice and resources focussing on lifestyle issues at the expense of the 'causes of the causes' (see Reflection on Practice 4.3) – in other words tackling

---

Reflection on Practice 4.3

If much of the evidence points to the social determinants of health being a key-driver for health outcomes and indeed health behaviours and practices, to what extent is a focus on health lifestyles ethical or effective? As a health promotion practitioner, perhaps working in a locality, how would you ensure that broader social, economic and environmental issues were being considered? Would you consider this within your remit and, if so, how would you seek to address some of the social determinants in your practice.

Also, consider that you *were* able as a practitioner to address the social determinants of health in your role. Given that everyone's health cannot be equal and the same, what levels of inequality would you be able to tolerate or accept?

manifestations of health inequalities (smoking, drinking, diet, exercise), rather than the fundamental causes (poverty, education, exclusion). Lifestyle drift is the inclination for policy that recognises the need to act on upstream social determinants only to drift downstream to focus on individual lifestyle factors (Popay et al., 2010). There are many reasons for health promoters to do this – lifestyle interventions are easier to devise, design and implement than 'upstream' interventions (Carey et al., 2016), as one example. Moreover, health is a political matter and policy decisions can frequently be underpinned by political timeliness (based on perceived short-term opportunities and political preferences), rather than credible research evidence (van de Goor et al., 2017).

A critique of empowerment

A constituent value within health promotion is empowerment and it has long been regarded as a crucial part of health promotion practice (Tilford et al., 2003). Some have even suggested that health promotion has become 'preoccupied' with empowerment but that this has caused a whole range of ambiguities that calls into question the ethical basis for espousing the approach (Buchanan, 2000). Buchanan writes:

> *The field of health promotion has joined the bandwagon of empowerment wholeheartedly, leaving its dark side unannounced and unexplored.*
>
> (Buchanan, 2000, p. 83)

One of the key challenges for health promotion practice has been the lack of consistency in regard to the understanding of what empowerment actually means. This has been a long-standing debate that will not be rehearsed here, but it is clear that the word has been used with casual abandon, with many health promotion projects and interventions (seemingly regardless of their function) aiming to 'empower' the populations they are working with (Woodall et al., 2012). Regardless of the definitional diversity, in essence empowerment is about marginalised groups gaining greater power and control over their circumstances. However, given that 'power' or resource is finite, resources being directed at some people can cause the displacement of power (disempowerment) from others due to competition for the same resources (Riger, 2002; Heritage and Dooris, 2009). Does this create ethical questions and indeed moral questions about who is deserving and undeserving? The notion of empowerment strategies for people in prison, for example, has never been an accepted pursuit in prison systems, even regarded as '*morally questionable and politically dangerous*' (The Aldridge Foundation and Johnson, 2008, p. 2). Yet, health promotion advocates claim that

---

Box 4.1   Empowerment with marginalised groups: an ethical challenge

If health promotion is to be implemented in prison settings, then understanding how empowerment can be fostered and the disempowerment of prisoners minimised is critical. Recent research has found that despite potential opportunity for people in prison to feel a greater sense of control and empowerment, this was completely eroded by the disempowering social and environmental factors that surrounded them. This included violence, humiliation and wider resource shortage. Even in very high-security prisons, people can feel empowered through having democratic rights and feeling able to influence change but the disempowering features of their prison life overshadowed these significantly (Woodall, 2020).

---

prisons should be supportive and empowering (de Viggiani et al., 2005; Woodall, 2020). Given the oppressive nature of many prison systems, is the notion of empowerment simply impossible with the raising expectations that it could be unethical (see Box 4.1).

Box 4.1 resonates with issues concerning individual empowerment and wider empowerment for structural change. Some argue that the original political and radical overtones of empowerment have been diluted within health promotion by concepts such as 'individual', 'psychological' or 'self' empowerment (Woodall et al., 2012). Individual empowerment alone has a limited impact on addressing health inequalities and may be illusory in that it does not lead to an increase in actual power or resources. In reality, empowerment simply at the individual level does little to influence social change:

Individual empowerment is not now, and never will be, the salvation of powerless groups. To attain social equality, power relations between 'haves,' 'have-a-littles,' and 'have-nots' must be transformed. This requires a change in the structure of power.

(Staples, 1990, p. 36)

There are ethical considerations in relation to empowerment, especially when empowerment is conceptualised as an outcome to be achieved. Empowerment itself may not be achievable for many – power will always sit with one group over another (Carter et al., 2012). Also, empowerment strategies may lead to communities or individuals to dominate others, or lead to communities demanding ineffective or harmful interventions (Carter et al., 2012). Buchanan's concern is that empowerment is a blunt approach that requires a more reasoned and nuanced, ethical stance:

> *In conclusion, my concern is that the push for empowerment teaches that exerting power is the best way to get what one wants. When health promotion specialists advocate and disseminate empowerment strategies, there is a corresponding depreciation of the value of reason, dialogue, and deliberation.*

(Buchanan, 2000, p. 83)

Does health promotion need a code of ethics to support practice?

Evidence suggests that most health promotion practitioners face individual and structural barriers to engaging productively with ethical frameworks for their practice, with most unaware of existing models (Blackford et al., 2022). That said, over 80% of health promoters do want a code of ethics to support them in their practice, feeling like this would strengthen, give credibility and legitimise their practice (Bull et al., 2012). An often-cited ethical code of practice comes from the Society of Health Education and Promotion Specialists (SHEPS, 2009), a now defunct group, that offers some practical guidance to navigating ethical challenges. There are, of course, a range of others (see the IUHPE). Many practitioners though, feel that an adaptation of the Ottawa Charter to help ethical decision-making would be most useful (Bull et al., 2012).

Whilst there is considerable appetite for a code of ethics from health promoters, the process of devising this would not be straightforward. It is likely that they would be too general and in reality, unable to provide specific guidance for specific situations. Conversely, they would have to be exceptionally detailed, leaving them completely impractical as tools for daily decision-making (Seedhouse, 2002).

As discussed in Chapter 2, the principles of autonomy (not doing anything that goes against a person's wishes), non-maleficence (not doing harm), beneficence (doing good) and justice (treating people equally and with respect) provide a useful starting point in relation to a framework for practice, but the debate on whether health promoters require an explicit code of practice or framework to guide their work continues (Sindall, 2002). At the very least, ethical theory and teaching should be incorporated into the health promotion curriculum and into training programmes for the current workforce (Sindall, 2002). This may provide practitioners with a greater understanding of ethical principles and therefore feel more confident to apply these within their daily practice. Reflection on Practice 4.4 explains this in more detail.

Reflection on Practice 4.4

David Seedhouse has been a prominent figure in addressing ethical issues and tensions in health promotion. Below are a list of questions, drawn from his ethical grid, that Seedhouse (2008) has suggested practitioners consider in their decision-making:

1 Central conditions in working for health
    a Am I creating autonomy in my clients, enabling them to direct their own lives?
    b Am I respecting the autonomy of my clients, whether or not I approve of their chosen direction?
    c Am I respecting all people as equal?
    d Do I work with people on the basis of needs first?
2 Key principles in working for health
    a Am I doing good and avoiding harm?
    b Am I telling the truth and keeping promises?
3 Consequences of ways of working for health
    a Will my action increase the individual good?
    b Will it increase the good of a particular group?
    c Will it increase the good of society?
    d Will I be acting for the good of myself?
4 External considerations in working for health
    a Are there any legal implications?
    b Is there a risk attached to the intervention?
    c Is the intervention the most effective and efficient action to take?
    d How certain is the evidence on which this intervention is based?
    e What are the views and wishes of those involved?
    f Can I justify my actions in terms of all this evidence?

There is a gap currently in relation to an agreed code of ethics. Given the ever-complex, fast-paced and dynamic global context and the implications of this for health and wellbeing it is perhaps timely to reinvigorate discussion on key principles for health promotion practice to ensure ethical reasoning has been given due consideration.

Summary

This chapter has highlighted a range of ethical dilemmas and challenges facing practitioners. These challenges are difficult to navigate and it is clear that many issues require careful consideration. Health promotion, as commonly conceptualised, is a discipline that seeks to achieve fairer and healthier communities. Intentions of health promoters are almost always laudable, but the chapter has shown a series of examples where damaging, unethical side-effects can result from poorly conceived interventions and in some cases, health promotion activity can create more problems than solutions. Ethics in health promotion has not received full attention, but evidence shows that practitioners would benefit from a code of practice to guide their decision-making. To date, however, a unified code has not been forthcoming.

Key points

- Health promotion practice has innumerable ethical tensions and challenges. This can vary from providing health communication, or to working in ways that are empowering.
- Serious consideration is needed in order to resolve some of the ethical challenges faced by practitioners.
- A code of practice to help health promoters navigate ethical dilemmas is in great demand, but a unified view on this has not been forthcoming.

Further reading

Blackford, K., Leavy, J., Taylor, J., Connor, E. and Crawford, G. (2022) Towards an ethics framework for Australian health promotion practitioners: An exploratory mixed methods study. *Health Promotion Journal of Australia*, 33, 71–82.
This paper provides up-to-date insight into the challenges and opportunities in relation to ethical issues facing health promoters. It calls for a stronger debate on the nature of ethics in health promotion and argues for an ethical framework to guide practical decision-making.
Carter, S. M., Cribb, A. and Allegrante, J. P. (2012) How to think about health promotion ethics. *Public Health Reviews*, 34, 1–24.
This paper covers a range of theoretical debates that have direct application to health promotion practice. The paper explores how to think ethically and calls for greater consideration and thought on health promotion ethics.
Le Fanu, J. (1994) *Preventionitis: the Exaggerated Claims of Health Promotion.* London, Social Affairs Unit.
This is certainly not a contemporary book, but its scathing critique of health promotion and the ethics of prevention is worth reading. It is a critical exploration of health promotion which, whilst some policy references are dated, still has a contemporary flavour with themes around vaccination and screening still being relevant.

References

Barić, L. (1992) Health promoting hospitals. *Journal of the Institute of Health Education*, 30, 141–148.

Beattie, A. (1991) Knowledge and control in health promotion: A test case for social policy and social theory. In: Gabe, J., Calnan, M. and Bury, M. (Eds.), *The Sociology of the Health Service*. London, Routledge.

Beauchamp, D. (1987) Life-style, public health and paternalism. In: Doxiadis, S. (Ed.), *Ethical Dilemmas in Health Promotion*. New York, John Wiley & Sons.

Becker, M.H. (1986) The tyranny of health promotion. *Public Health Reviews*, 14, 15–23.

Belsky, J., Melhuish, E., Barnes, J., Leyland, A.H. and Romaniuk, H. (2006) Effects of Sure Start local programmes on children and families: Early findings from a quasi-experimental, cross sectional study. *BMJ*, 332, 1476.

Blackford, K., Leavy, J., Taylor, J., Connor, E. and Crawford, G. (2022) Towards an ethics framework for Australian health promotion practitioners: An exploratory mixed methods study. *Health Promotion Journal of Australia*, 33, 71–82.

Brown, R.C. (2018) Resisting moralisation in health promotion. *Ethical Theory and Moral Practice*, 21, 997–1011.

Brown, R.C., Maslen, H. and Savulescu, H. (2019) Against moral responsibilisation of health: Prudential responsibility and health promotion. *Public Health Ethics*, 12, 114–129.

Buchanan, D.R. (2000) *An Ethic for Health Promotion*. New York, Oxford University Press.

Bull, T., Riggs, E. and Nchogu, S.N. (2012) Does health promotion need a Code of Ethics? Results from an IUHPE mixed method survey. *Global Health Promotion*, 19, 8–20.

Cardona, B. (2020) The pitfalls of personalization rhetoric in time of health crisis: COVID-19 pandemic and cracks on neoliberal ideologies. *Health Promotion International*, 36, 714–721.

Carey, G., Malbon, E., Crammond, B., Pescud, M. and Baker, P. (2016) Can the sociology of social problems help us to understand and manage 'lifestyle drift'? *Health Promotion International*, 1–7. http://dx.doi.org/10.1093/heapro/dav116

Carter, S.M., Cribb, A. and Allegrante, J.P. (2012) How to think about health promotion ethics. *Public Health Reviews*, 34, 1–24.

Catford, J. (2004) Health promotion's record card: How principled are we 20 years on? *Health Promotion International*, 19, 1–3.

Clarke, K. (2006) Childhood, parenting and early intervention: A critical examination of the Sure Start national programme. *Critical Social Policy*, 26, 699–721.

Crawford, R. (1980) Healthism and the medicalization of everyday life. *International Journal of Health Services*, 10, 365–388.

Cross, R., Davis, S. and O'Neil, I. (2017) *Health Communication: Theoretical and Critical Perspectives*. Cambridge, Polity.

de Viggiani, N., Orme, J., Powell, J. and Salmon, D. (2005) New arrangements for prison health care provide an opportunity and a challenge for primary care trusts. *British Medical Journal*, 330, 918.

Demirtaş-Madran, H.A. (2021) Accepting restrictions and compliance with recommended preventive behaviors for COVID-19: A discussion based on the key approaches and current research on fear appeals. *Frontiers in Psychology*, 12, 1–15.

Department of Health (1992) *The Health of the Nation: A Strategy for Health in England*. London: HMSO.

Dooris, M. and Hunter, D.J. (2007) Organisations and settings for promoting public health. In: Lloyd, C.E., Handsley, S., Douglas, J., Earle, S. and Spurr, S. (Eds.), *Policy and Practice in Promoting Public Health*. London, Sage.

Fitzgerald, F.T. (1994) The tyranny of health. *The New England Journal of Medicine*, 3, 196–198.

Green, J., Cross, R., Woodall, J. and Tones, K. (2019) *Health Promotion. Planning and Strategies*. London, Sage.

Green, L.W., Poland, B.D. and Rootman, I. (2000) The settings approach to health promotion. In: Poland, B.D., Green, L.W. and Rootman, I. (Eds.), *Settings for Health Promotion. Linking Theory and Practice*. Thousand Oaks, Sage.

Gugglberger, L. (2018) Can health promotion also do harm? *Health Promotion International*, 33, 557–560.

Guttman, N. (2017) *Ethical Issues in Health Promotion and Communication Interventions, Oxford Research Encyclopaedias: Communication*. Oxford, Oxford University Press.

Heffner, J., Vives, M.-L. and FeldmanHall, O. (2021) Emotional responses to prosocial messages increase willingness to self-isolate during the COVID-19 pandemic. *Personality and Individual Differences*, 170, 110420.

Heritage, Z. and Dooris, M. (2009) Community participation and empowerment in Healthy Cities. *Health Promotion International*, 24, 45–55.

Hubley, J., Copeman, J. and Woodall, J. (2021) *Practical Health Promotion*. Cambridge, Polity Press.

Le Fanu, J. (1994) *Preventionitis: the Exaggerated Claims of Health Promotion*. London, Social Affairs Unit.

Marmot, M. (1996) The social pattern of health and disease. In: Blane, D., Brunner, E. and Wilkinson, R. (Eds.), *Health and Social Organization: Towards a Health Policy for the Twenty-First Century*. London, Routledge.

Marmot, M. (2002) The influence of income on health: Views of an epidemiologist. *Health Affairs*, 21, 31–46.

Marmot, M. (2010) Fair society, healthy lives. The Marmot Review. Strategic Review of Health Inequalities in England Post-2010. London, The Marmot Review.

Marmot, M., Allen, J., Boyce, T., Goldblatt, P. and Morrison, J. (2020a) *Health Equity in England: the Marmot Review 10 Years on*. London, Institute of Health Equity.

Marmot, M., Allen, J., Goldblatt, P., Herd, E. and Morrison, J. (2020b) Build back fairer: The COVID-19 marmot review. The Pandemic, Socioeconomic and Health Inequalities in England. London, UCL.

Marmot, M., Friel, S., Bell, R., Houweling, T.A. and Taylor, S. (2008) Closing the gap in a generation: Health equity through action on the social determinants of health. *The Lancet*, 372, 1661–1669.

Nettleton, S. (1995) *The Sociology of Health & Illness.* Cambridge, Polity Press.

Newall, P.W.S., Weiss-Cohen, L., Singmann, H., Walasek, L. and Ludvig, E.A. (2022) Impact of the "when the fun stops, stop" gambling message on online gambling behaviour: A randomised, online experimental study. *The Lancet Public Health*, 7, e437–e446.

Petticrew, M., Maani, N., Pettigrew, L., Rutter, H. and Van Schalkwyk, M.C. (2020) Dark nudges and sludge in big alcohol: Behavioral economics, cognitive biases, and alcohol industry corporate social responsibility. *The Milbank Quarterly*, 98, 1290–1328.

Popay, J., Whitehead, M. and Hunter, D.J. (2010) Injustice is killing people on a large scale—but what is to be done about it? *Journal of Public Health*, 32, 148–149.

Riger, S. (2002) What's wrong with empowerment. In: Revenson, T.A., D'augelli, A.R., French, S.E., Hughes, D., Livert, D.E., Seidman, E., Shinn, M. and Yoshikawa, H. (Eds.), *Quarter Century of Community Psychology: Readings from the American Journal of Community Psychology.* New York, Kluwer Academic/Plenum.

Rintoul, A. (2022) Can slogans prevent gambling harm? *The Lancet Public Health*, 7, e394–e395.

Rutter, M. (2006) Is Sure Start an effective preventive intervention? *Child and Adolescent Mental Health*, 11, 135–141.

Scriven, A. (2017) *Promoting Health: a Practical Guide* London. Bailliere Tindall.

Seedhouse, D. (2002) Commitment to health: A shared ethical bond between professions. *Journal of Interprofessional Care*, 16, 249–260.

Seedhouse, D. (2008) *Ethics: the Heart of Health Care.* Chichester, John Wiley & Sons.

SHEPS (2009) *A Framework for Ethical Health Promotion.* Wales, SHEPS.

Sindall, C. (2002) Does health promotion need a code of ethics? *Health Promotion International*, 17, 201–203.

Skrabanek, P. (1990) Why is preventive medicine exempted from ethical constraints? *Journal of Medical Ethics*, 16, 187–190.

Smith, C. (2000) Healthy prisons: A contradiction in terms? *The Howard Journal of Criminal Justice*, 39, 339–353.

South, J. and Tilford, S. (2000) Perceptions of research and evaluation in health promotion practice and influences on activity. *Health Education Research*, 15, 729–741.

Speller, V. (2006) Developing healthy settings. In: Macdowall, W., Bonell, C. and Davis, M. (Eds.), *Health Promotion Practice.* Maidenhead, Open University Press.

Staples, L.H. (1990) Powerful ideas about empowerment. *Administration in Social Work*, 14, 29–42.

The Aldridge Foundation & Johnson, M. (2008) *The User Voice of the Criminal Justice System.* London, The Aldridge Foundation.

Tilford, S., Green, J. and Tones, K. (2003) *Values, Health Promotion and Public Health.* Leeds, Centre for Health Promotion Research, Leeds Metropolitan University.

van de Goor, I., Hämäläinen, R.-M., Syed, A., Juel Lau, C., Sandu, P., Spitters, H., Eklund Karlsson, L., Dulf, D., Valente, A., Castellani, T. and Aro, A.R. (2017)

Determinants of evidence use in public health policy making: Results from a study across six EU countries. *Health Policy*, 121, 273–281.

van Schalkwyk, M.C.I., Maani, N., McKee, M., Thomas, S., Knai, C. and Petticrew, M. (2021) "When the Fun Stops, Stop": An analysis of the provenance, framing and evidence of a 'responsible gambling' campaign. *PLOS ONE*, 16, e0255145.

WHO (1986) Ottawa Charter for health promotion. *Health Promotion*, 1, iii–v.

Williams, G. (1985) Health promotion—caring concern or slick salesmanship? *Journal of the Institute of Health Education*, 23, 26–33.

Williams, O. and Fullagar, S. (2019) Lifestyle drift and the phenomenon of 'citizen shift' in contemporary UK health policy. *Sociology of Health & Illness*, 41, 20–35.

Wilson, L.C., Farley, A. and Horton, S.F. (2022) The impact of victim blaming and locus of control on mental health outcomes among female sexual assault survivors. *Violence Against Women*, 28, 3785–3800.

Woodall, J. (2020) Health promotion co-existing in a high-security prison context: A documentary analysis. *International Journal of Prisoner Health*, http://dx.doi.org/10.1108/IJPH-09-2019-0047.

Woodall, J. and Cross, R. (2021) *Essentials of Health Promotion*. London, Sage.

Woodall, J. and Rowlands, S. (2020) Professional practice. In: Cross, R., Foster, S., O'neil, I., Rowlands, S., Woodall, J. and Warwick-Booth, L. (Eds.), *Health Promotion: Global Principles and Practice*. London, CABI.

Woodall, J., Warwick-Booth, L. and Cross, R. (2012) Has empowerment lost its power? *Health Education Research*, 27, 742–745.

5 Ethics in health promotion research

Introduction

This chapter explores ethics in relation to health promotion research. This chapter draws upon previous discussions about ethics as a key concern for health promotion, and ethics in practice to consider how key principles from these areas should be applied and used when researching health promotion. We discuss the key ethical principles that researchers need to be aware of as detailed by ethical committees, and then specifically apply these to health promotion research. This chapter therefore considers issues that health promotion researchers have to be aware of and contend with, beyond simple ethical approval. This chapter details doing research *with* people, not on them or to them, in keeping with the values of health promotion discussed earlier in the book. The chapter provides discussion about participatory, creative methods of research as well as methods which privilege people's voices and experiences such as qualitative approaches to research, discussing the ways in which these methods sit with the core values of the discipline. There is consideration and discussion of the power dynamic in the research process, as well as more specifically within research relationships and reflection about how to minimise this, for example, by using inclusive methods. The chapter contains examples case studies which adopt anti-mainstream approaches such as feminism. This chapter informs the reader about how to do health promotion research in more ethical ways.

By the end of this chapter, the reader should be able to:

- Understand how to apply the ethical principles of research to health promotion studies;
- Identify the importance of using methods to privilege people's voices and experiences;
- Understand the importance of doing research with people, rather than on them or to them, by using inclusive anti-mainstream approaches.

DOI: 10.4324/9781003308317-5

The importance of research ethics

All research, including health promotion studies are governed by ethical principles and associated scrutiny by bodies of approval such as ethics committees. Previous historical abuses of power during research, led to the development of a field of ethics specifically applied to data collection, offering general guidance about suitable ways of working (Warwick-Booth et al., 2021). Historically there have been many abuses and misuses of power during research studies, where participants have been physically or psychologically harmed as a consequence. Research conducted in the past may be defined as unethical when measured against contemporary ethical standards, but it is also important to note that even well-intentioned research can cause harm without meaning to do so. For example, some clinical trials testing new drugs and treatment, can result in unexpected side effects despite the ethical measures that have been put in place to govern them. Indeed, there are many factors affecting the success of clinical trial (Fogel, 2018). Some studies may also result in psychological harm, for example the infamous psychological study conducted by Milgram (1963), which tested the ways in which people responded to authority by being obedient is discussed in the literature as unethical in terms of the potential psychological harm it resulted in Warwick-Booth et al. (2021). Therefore, research ethics guidelines and review processes are intended to work as a mechanism to prevent harm, and to ensure that research is conducted appropriately and morally.

Principles guiding research ethics

Research methods literature indicates that there are some key ethical principles that all researchers need to consider within their own practice of research. In addition to these general guidelines, institutions such as universities and health services also have their own specific standards detailing the principles that researchers are expected to adhere to. Table 5.1. details the standard ethical principles which need to be considered in all studies.

Table 5.1 details standard ethics principles related to research studies, and compares them to general ethical guidelines for health promotion practice. Health promotion as a discipline has specific values underpinning ethical practice (as discussed in earlier chapters) whilst public health research is additionally guided by ethics review processes (Klinger et al., 2020).Samuel et al. (2022) also discuss the concept of ethical preparedness as a requirement for both practice and research. They argue that ethical decision making needs to be understood as a behaviour, applied across

Table 5.1 Standard ethical principles, and their relevance to health promotion research

Ethical principles of research	Health promotion ethics (IHPE, 2022)
Protection from harm, also commonly discussed as do no harm. In each study that researchers conduct, they need to pay attention to the potential harm that the work might cause for participants as well as researchers. This includes physical, social and emotional harm. Steps should be taken to avoid doing harm, or to minimise it, if it is not possible to completely control it. Usually ethical committees require researchers to conduct a risk assessment for each study that they do, and to pay attention to relevant health and safety guidelines.	The IHPE (2022) position statement on ethics mentions the importance of managing harm in health promotion practice, as well as conducting risk assessments.
Participant information should be provided to ensure informed consent (see related discussion below). Information about each research study needs to be provided to anyone who is interested in taking part, so that they know what the study is about, what is expected of them, and what the researchers will do with the data. Potential participants can ask questions about the study, so they need to be made aware of their rights to questioning. This is standard practice unless the research is covert (hidden) from participants who remain unaware that they are being studied.	The IHPE (2022) position statement on ethics discusses the need for clear communication practices, as well as open discussion of ethical issues in health promotion practice.
Informed consent is another principle and is a term used to describe the processes that researchers use to ensure that participants are fully aware of the research process and consent to involvement following discussion and the provision of information about the study, and what it is aiming to achieve. Standard ways of achieving informed consent, involve researchers producing written information sheets about the study and what it involves, as well as consent forms for participants to complete. In some instances, consent is recorded verbally, and information provision is adapted to meet participant needs for example, if the study population has low literacy levels.	IPHE (2022) practice guidelines note the need for clear communication methods, and clear discussion of ethical issues.
Anonymity is an ethical principle that researchers are expected to adhere to. Any individual who takes part in a research study	The IHPE (2022) ethical principles, discuss the need to consider potential

(Continued)

Table 5.1 (Continued)

Ethical principles of research	Health promotion ethics (IHPE, 2022)
should not be identifiable in the research results, such as reports, presentations and other dissemination formats. Researchers usually achieve anonymity by allocating participants different names, or labels in the presentation of the data. However, if the study uses innovative and creative methods for example, include photographs, films, poems and plays then anonymity may not be achievable. Each dissemination format raises different challenges in terms of anonymity.	harm (as noted above), therefore if anonymity is not certain, there may be additional harms to take into account.
Confidentiality. Those who take part in research should be made aware that what they say is confidential and not linked to them, in line with the principle of anonymity described above. However, in some instances researchers have a duty of care to report potential harms, if safeguarding issues are identified during the research process which overrides the principle of confidentiality.	This principle is in line with IHPE (2022) guidance to managing risk.
The right to withdraw. Participants can change their mind about taking part in the research even after signing the consent forms, and starting to provide data. So they can take part in an interview and during that, decide to no longer contribute. However, once research results are published withdrawal is no longer possible.	This is in line with the ethical practice of working in an empowering manner, encouraging but not forcing public participation, as well as considering ethical issues when promoting health (IHPE, 2022).
Care of participants is an essential ethical principle, underpinned by respect. Researchers are expected not to exploit participants, to work in respectful relationships and to protect community values.	This is again in line with working in an enabling manner, involving listening to participants' views (which may differ) in a positive way, as per IHPE (2022) ethical health promotion guidance.
Data protection is essential in all research projects. Secure data storage has to be a given, with any raw data (e.g. interview recordings and transcripts) not using real names or any other identifying information. Electronic data (recordings, scanned forms, notes) should be stored within password-protected systems or encrypted. Any paper copies of information should be locked away.	This is again about management of risk, and protecting people from harm, in line with IHPE (2022) recommendations.

**Reflection on Practice 5.1: Applying principles
in research practice**

Which of the key ethical principles discussed in Table 5.1 are
more difficult to apply than others, when doing health promotion
research?

The IHPE (2022) principles for ethical health promotion
practice outlines the importance of participation, saying that it
is crucial. Participation as a key ethical value underpinning health
promotion practice has been discussed in detail in earlier chapters
(see Chapter 1). However, in most research studies public participation in the design of the work before ethical review stage is
not standard practice. Participation in research also takes varying
forms, and is understood differently by researchers. Staley and
Elliot (2017) discuss how lay people's ethics-related contributions
are also often excluded from research reports.

- In what ways might people be excluded from ethical
  conversations?
- What might this mean in terms of health promotion research
  on key disciplinary issues such as health inequalities, and the
  social determinants of health?
- How might you, as a health promotion researcher, need to
  consider how your own research practices in a critical manner?
  For example, adhering to standard ethical guidelines may still
  be problematic in various, differing contexts.

both research and practice. Reflection on Practice 5.1 offers questions to
stimulate thinking about being ethically prepared during research practice.

Having reflected on the challenges of applying health promotion values to research, and the complexities of using principles in practice, it
is important to note that ethical approaches should be adapted for different contexts, studies and participants (Kara, 2018, p. 9). Similarly,
Al Tajir (2018) notes that whilst traditional ethical principles should be
applied to public health research, the nature of the discipline itself raises
broader ethical challenges because health promotion involves working
to gather data during public health emergencies, disease outbreaks and
natural disasters – all of which raise additional complexities associated
with the ethical conduct of research.

Research studies and their ethical approaches are assessed by committees, for example within university settings, healthcare (NHS), or via

other professional bodies. Anyone undertaking a study is required to seek ethical approval, before they start to gather any data. The principles outlined in Table 5.1 need to therefore be considered and applied to each research study that is conducted. Al Tajir (2018) argues that conducting research responsibly is about moving beyond just understanding ethical guidance and principles, because real-life situations require further ethical scrutiny especially in situations where immediate action is needed due to a public health crisis. Therefore, balancing potential progress and harm is an ongoing issue for ethical public health research. Indeed, ethical committee approval, whilst necessary is just the start of working towards ethical research practice.

Kara (2018) is critical about research ethics processes and associated committee approval mechanisms. She argues that they tend to focus upon data-gathering only at the beginning of a project, and therefore do not acknowledge that ethical principles need to be applied in a continuous manner throughout all studies. The process of gaining ethical approval through committees, she argues, pushes researchers into form filling (consent forms, data storage documents), rather than encouraging them to reflect on the realities of what ethical practice actually means during fieldwork (Kara, 2017). Researchers need to consider consent in terms of how it will be obtained, once, or in a more negotiated ongoing manner, as well as what form is most appropriate in each project (verbal or written). Flicker et al. (2010) also suggest that communal consent needs consideration in community-based research. Kara (2017) then highlights that the economic pressures on researchers working in funded environments are an important consideration for health promoters, because attempting to achieve social justice through research is difficult in time-limited, and costed models of data collection (Kara, 2018). Finally, Kara (2017, 2018), and others (Garcia et al., 2013; Smith, 2013; Rix et al., 2018) note that ethical principles and processes tend to be Euro-Western, underpinned by colonial privileges, which are unjust for Indigenous populations, and unable to tackle structural inequalities. Ultimately accounting for context is essential when applying research principles in health promotion research, given its global focus, as there is an on-going need to decolonialise ethical approaches (Kara, 2018), as detailed in Case Study 5.1.

In addition to considering cultural challenges underpinning ethical health promotion research, given the nature of health promotion as a discipline, many research projects involve collecting data from vulnerable or marginalised communities in general life rather than in public health emergency situations (Al Tajir, 2018). Conducting research with communities deemed to be vulnerable and/or marginalised understandably requires additional consideration of participant needs in an ethical manner to ensure adequate protection, and doing no harm. Defining

Case study 5.1   Indigenous research methods and ethics

Kara (2018) in writing about research ethics in the real world criticises current ethical practices, and methods for being too Eurocentric. She argues that Indigenous research methods pre-date those used in Europe, and the global north by thousands of years, and are underpinned by local contextual knowledge. However, the academic literature on research from the global north fails to discuss this, and tends to adopt a position in which Eurocentric versions of ethical practice are assumed to be a world-wide set of rules. She argues that there is much to be learned from Indigenous practices, defining these as:

1 Relational accountability – the researcher is accountable to everyone and everything connected to the research. This encompasses a much wider view than ethical committees take as it includes ancestors, land and on-going relationships with research participants;
2 Communality of knowledge – no one individual can own knowledge because it is relational, and should be reciprocally exchanged for the benefit of all involved.

Kara (2018) argues that researchers from the global north are not able to adopt these principles in the same way as Indigenous communities because of cultural differences, noting that European researchers have historically tended to extract information and then use it for their own benefit, which is abusive. There needs to be, in her view, a move to working together more collaboratively to understand, develop and co-produce ethical guides that are workable for all, starting with English speaking colonialist advantage being addressed.

marginalised and/or vulnerable participants is open to much debate, but can include populations who have low literacy levels, communities with limited economic resources, people who are not able to make decisions about consenting to taking part in research, young people and those with learning disabilities (Shallwani and Mohammed, 2007). This list is not exhaustive, and we are not suggesting that these groups of people should be excluded from research projects, simply because they are considered to be vulnerable, and therefore more ethically challenging.

However, conducting research for health promotion, often means that such groups will be part of studies due to the need for promoting equity and social justice (see Chapter 1). Warwick-Booth et al. (2021) argue that in researching these groups, attention has to be given to the characteristics of participants in each instance. For example, when working with children in health promotion research, access has to be negotiated at multiple levels for example, with the adults who control children's lives and the contexts in which they exist (i.e. schools). Children's right to give informed consent cannot be assumed as parental consent may additionally be required. Confidentiality and anonymity also need further consideration when working with marginalised communities as identities are more likely to be disclosed or inferred within such contexts. In such instances, are all participants aware of any limits to confidentiality? Researchers need to consider issues such as blurred boundaries in relation to anonymity, whilst balancing being inclusive with protecting participant identity and rights to data access (Flicker et al., 2010).

Health promotion research topics also need to be given critical attention, as they are often linked to moral dimensions such as good and bad choices (see Chapter 4), or individualised notions of problems which are stigmatised. Pause (2017) writes about the ethics of fat stigma in public health, caused by the neo-liberal framing of responsibility in which people are labelled as lazy, the cause of their own fatness through their choices, and behaviours and therefore flawed in character. Conducting research on this topic, and other stigmatised subjects relevant to contemporary health promotion practice, raises additional ethical challenges as the work should be done in a way to minimise any stigma in line with the public health values, whilst doing no harm. Conducting research on any sensitive, stigmatised topic is likely to do some harm, in terms of emotional responses among participants at the very least. Indeed, researchers may also experience a range of emotions, therefore ethical practice should also consider their health needs. Emotional labour for researchers is underreported in the literature, though work is now emerging and there are several ways in which to support researcher wellbeing. Warwick-Booth et al. (2023) note the importance of self-care for researchers, describing their own strategies which include debrief, writing reflective notes and self-care. They argue that ongoing discussion of researcher wellbeing is needed in health promotion research work, given the nature of the disciplines focus on inequalities and disadvantage. Similarly, Delderfield (2018) outlines the need for researchers to employ a myriad of strategies in support of their own emotional processing. Finally, Hall (2019, p. 161) also uses the term 'emotional magnitude', to describe the need for researchers to recognise the emotional impact of their findings, and to therefore consider how to communicate these sensitively.

Health promotion research also tends to be conducted within community settings, and so is community-based, raising ethical considerations beyond the level of the individual. The ethical principles outlined in Table 5.1 are more focussed on individual level protections. For example, can anonymity always be ensured in small-scale community-based studies where people know each other very well? Questions such as this, and poor ethical practices when conducting research have led to the development of specific ethical codes which pay attention to community level research. For example, Indigenous communities have developed their own ethical guides in response to their dissatisfaction with the ways in which research has been done to them (as discussed earlier in Case Study 5.1). Examples include the Te Ara Tika, Guidelines for Māori Research Ethics, from New Zealand, and the San Code of Research Ethics from South Africa. The Centre for Social Justice and Community Action, Durham University (2012) also published broad guidance for researchers conducting community-based participatory research.

All research raises ethical challenges, but the distinctiveness of health promotion research requires further analysis. Woodall et al. (2018b) describe how health promotion research is defined by its focus on real world issues, its values, its expansive methodological toolkit and the ways in which professionals relinquish control. These considerations have led researchers to do their work in ways that try to empower participants involved in the research process, in line with disciplinary values. Much health promotion research involves doing research *with* people, not on them or to them, and involves in some instances participatory, creative methods of research.

Doing research ethically with people

Conducting health promotion research in communities with people, can be argued to be more ethical than traditional research studies, such as the Milgram (1963) experiment referred to at the start of this chapter, because this and other experiments caused harm (Armstrong et al., 2011). Working with people, and involving them is seen to be more inclusive, empowering and fairer in terms of power sharing, depending on the approach taken. There are a number of ways to work with people when doing research alongside them, as Woodall et al. (2018a) argue, health promotion researchers have an expansive methodological toolkit. For example, participatory research aligns with health promotion values and is used globally, and can take a variety of forms including co-productive approaches, and peer research work (Warwick-Booth et al., 2021); inclusive research has been applied to communities experiencing learning disabilities (Nind, 2017); creative methods encourage participation and representation of voice (Kara, 2020) and some research aims to be transformative by attempting to tackle social inequalities, and associated marginalisation (Kara, 2018; Warwick-Booth et al., 2023). These approaches, though different, share commonalities in their intention to work with and for people as part of the research process. Case Study 5.2 provides an example of feminist research intended to support social change in England, underpinned by health promotion values.

Case Study 5.2   Ethical feminist research for social change

Feminist research is a broad church, but is tied together by the intention to research gender through a critical, and anti-mainstream stance. Feminist methods sit well with the values that underpin health promotion as they are about questioning structural inequalities, advocating on behalf of marginalised women to ensure that their lived experiences are represented, challenging existing power dynamics and mainstream approaches, which in this instance mean male, positivist biases in research.

Feminist approaches to research have much to offer health promotion as a discipline, and in using such methods over a long period of time (a decade), Warwick-Booth et al. (2023) reflect upon their value in giving voice to women who are defined as seldomly heard such as those experiencing domestic abuse, and multiple complex needs. By using creative, participatory methods such as creative storyboards, metaphors and peer research approaches, research can empower participants. Co-production principles allow for a more flexible and inclusive approach to data generation, and taking part in research can itself be transformational.

However, despite the positives of this type of research work, caution is still required as funding agencies have agendas about evidence, research takes place in cultural contexts in which dominant social norms underpin social life, and power dynamics still exist despite researcher attempts to minimise these. Academics are often in privileged positions by the nature of their educational background, position and status. They also bring their own identities with them to the research process, so need to be aware of their positionality. The nature of feminist research related to vulnerabilities is also full of emotions for both the researchers and the researched, which raises further ethical challenge about to manage these, not only during data collection but also once this has been completed.

Adapted from Warwick-Booth et al. (2023).

Despite well-intentioned researchers, who aim to work with people, rather than doing research to them, there are many complexities that are associated with this type of work, as is often involves complicated relationships, power sharing, partnerships and blurred roles (Warwick-Booth et al., 2021). Indeed, each method that is used to gather data in health promotion research is likely to need tailored ethical considerations, particularly those in which participation is considered appropriate and more ethical. Guidelines on participatory research often suggest equal participation as ethical, however these fail to recognise existing inequalities and divisions within community settings. Flicker at al. (2010) therefore suggest that there are rarely right or wrong answers to challenging ethical issues, rather that reflection is always needed throughout the lifetime of any research project, a stance increasingly noted in the literature, associated with ongoing methodological developments.

There has been much development in methodological innovations for research methods within health promotion, as well as across other

Table 5.2 Example ethical considerations when using different methods

Method of data collection	Ethical questions
Traditional methods, applied with marginalised groups	Do written documents such as information sheets and consent forms work effectively in communities that have low literacy levels? Tamariz et al. (2013) argue that low health literacy also impairs participation in informed consent processes.
	How do researchers also effectively recognise and reward participant time? Is it now considered more ethical to offer incentives such as vouchers and travel expenses, but debates continue about how to fairly calculate these (London et al., 2012). In addition, should children be rewarded in the same way as adults are (Sime, 2008)?
	What about research in sensitive settings, with vulnerable populations? Woodall (2010) reflects on the ethics of conducting health promotion research in prison settings, debating the extent to which informed consent can be achieved with captive participants. Given that such participants are powerless, and are inclined to participate to pass time, researchers must take extra care to ensure that ethical practices are met. Robust ethical practice in his research practice included providing information in varying formats, outlining the limitations to achieving confidentiality and ensuring that post-research support was available to manage potential mental health issues arising. Researcher self-care was also carefully managed through the development a specific strategy.

(Continued)

Table 5.2 (Continued)

Method of data collection	Ethical questions
Methods where participants may be more identifiable for example, film, photographs, drama.	Some research methods mean that participants are more identifiable by their very nature. Shaw (2016) argues that researchers need to ask if participants are comfortable being filmed and seeing themselves on film? Do all participants fully understand the implications of filming, and therefore what they are consenting to? Are all participants able to express emotions to researchers, and convey the ways in which such approaches to data collection make them feel? There are many more questions which need negotiation when using creative methods, including film (Shaw, 2021). Indeed, tensions may arise when researchers are trying to ensure ethical practice, participant safety, enjoyment and the creation of research products (Gubrium et al., 2014). Dynamic consent is therefore needed (Black et al., 2018). In using photovoice (conducting research with pictures) with children to engage them, Abma et al. (2022) reported many ethical dilemmas in their health promotion research. For example, who is in control of the outcome? What should photos be used for – voice, or representation? Who decides which individuals are visible in the pictures? Research studies using drama and role-play methods can be made more ethical, less sensitive and resolve identity by creating fictional characters. This worked well when researching HIV in Vietnam (Black et al., 2018).
Online methods	The COVID-19 pandemic and associated lock-downs in many locations, led to much face-to-face working transitioning into online work, creating ethical debates. Online methods may not work as well with vulnerable and marginalised communities, and must be adapted in each application (Warwick-Booth and Coan, 2022). In some instances, researchers may choose to exclude groups from participation if they are unsure of how to apply ethical rules for example, not doing research with children online (Facca et al., 2020).

disciplines. New methods of data collection are often described as important for enabling and representing marginalised voices (Kindon, 2003), particularly in the global south (Black et al., 2018), but ethical questions always need to be addressed. Again, there are ethical codes of conduct available related to visual methods (see https://visualsociology.org/) and guidance for researchers using the internet to gather data (https://aoir.org/), as each of these methods raises different ethical challenges. Table 5.2 provides some example ethical questions for consideration, related to a range of methods.

Table 5.2 provides several examples of general ethical questions for consideration in health promotion research, considering a range of different methods. However, there are of course more methods, huge variation in the topics likely to be explored and many more ethical considerations to pay attention to. For example, if using enhanced interview techniques such as a walking interview, this may create a more naturalistic conversation, give participants more agency but data collection in a public place, raises concerns about confidentiality as well as other challenges (Adekoya and Guse, 2020). This chapter has therefore constantly reinforced the idea of ethical practice varying according to each health promotion research project. Table 5.3. provides some examples of ethical dilemmas, and their resolution from our own practice, again illustrating the need for situated ethical approaches, applied to each health promotion study.

Table 5.2 provides illustrative examples of how ethical issues were debated and to some extent resolved, in several health promotion research projects. As each study raises different ethical challenges, transparent discussion of how these are dealt with are important for health promoters conducting research in practice, to ensure ongoing learning.

Due to the challenges identified in Table 5.2 and more broadly throughout this chapter, some researchers (Kawulich and Ogletree, 2012; Kara, 2018; Warwick-Booth et al., 2021) argue that there are additional ethical considerations to be made when working to do research with people, irrespective of the chosen model. Banks et al. (2013, p. 266) make a case for using 'everyday ethics', which they define as the constant negotiation of ethical issues during the lifetime of the research project. In addition, Banks et al. (2013) mention the importance of taking into account contextual issues for each research project. Health promotion researchers should be working with ethical sensitivity, to identify ethical challenges in each project and community, as it may be inappropriate for local researchers to work on certain types of research projects (Warwick-Booth et al., 2021). In Uganda, for example, it may not be appropriate to use local people to collect data on sensitive and stigmatised issues such as HIV/AIDS, as using peer researchers in such work is likely to lead to further stigma, and therefore harm (Cornwall and Jewkes, 1995). Therefore, it is essential to reflect upon ethical issues in the context of each health promotion research study, as detailed in Box 5.2.

Table 5.3 Health promotion research ethics applied in practice

Research study	Ethics in practice
Inspiring Change Evaluation Working to research experiences of homelessness, and multiple associated support needs in the north of England, Woodall et al. (2016) fore fronted service user views at the heart of this service evaluation. Training homeless service users as peer researchers, to undertake one-to-one interviews with others enabled wider reach into service user experiences.	The evaluation received standard ethical approval through university procedures Several traditional ethical principles were relevant to this work, and so were applied in practice. For example, informed consent and anonymity. The training of peer researchers also included detail on ethical principles, staying safe, gaining consent and doing no harm. Attention was paid to the ways in which taking part may harm both the peer researchers and the participants (Woodall et al., 2018a). Working as peer researchers was beneficial for those who adopted this role as they described improved confidence, raised self-esteem and transferable skills from being involved. This is therefore an ethical approach to research, linked to health promotion goals as it can empower peer researchers (Woodall et al., 2016). Peer researchers also received compensation for their time, and efforts through shopping vouchers – this is considered to be good practice in such work (Terry, 2016).
COVID-19 Grants Scheme Evaluation Warwick-Booth and Coan (2022) were commissioned to qualitatively evaluate a local authority response to COVID-19, during the legally enforceable lock-down periods in England. A key component of the response focussed upon reaching communities who were vulnerable and marginalised across one city in the north of England, because these groups were more likely to be socially isolated, have less access to services, support and up-to-date public health information about staying safe, and vaccinations.	Ethical approval for the evaluation was granted through standard University processes. Data collection had to be completed online due to lock-down rules. Ethical principles were applied, but some adaptation was required due to the online nature of the work. Warwick-Booth and Coan (2022) describe how they started using 'usual' practice, and then worked to adapt their approach because traditional ethical guidelines are not always sufficient when working online (Lavorgna and Sugiura, 2020). They used a tiered approach to gaining consent, seeking written consent via email first, and then moving to verbal consent where needed. Data collection tools were varied to allow participant choice (telephone interviews, MS Teams, Zoom, Skype, an online survey) but where participants were filmed during data collection (Skype, Teams and Zoom) only verbally recorded content was saved for analysis to increase anonymity. Warwick-Booth and Coan (2022) also acknowledge their attempts to offer care for participants' well-being given the nature of the evaluation topic, but reflect that they did not have the same non-verbal cues to observe distress, due to the online context in which data collection took place.

Reflection on Practice 5.2: Thinking about your own approach to ethical research as a health promoter

a Long et al. (2016) provide a list of questions for researchers who are using participatory approaches, so that they can reflect upon their own ethical stance in relation to their practices. These questions, are useful for you to consider when you work in any type of health promotion research, using all methods: What are the implications for research when communities are divided?

b Researchers often wear different hats for example, organiser, teacher, consultant, funder) so consider what issues this raises?

c What do you think are appropriate ways to credit and reward community members who work on research projects alongside you?

d How can research be done so that it promotes lasting benefits for the community?

Paying attention to your own characteristics and how these might influence your view of ethics in practice is also important here. For example, how might your identity influence your view of what is ethical practice? Are you privileged in any way? What is your status in society and how might this determine your research practice, especially your ethical stance?

Summary

This chapter has explored and debated ethics in relation to health promotion research, particularly focussing on ethical ways of researching health promotion. The chapter discussed the key ethical principles that researchers need to be aware of, and then specifically applied these to health promotion research topics, contexts and practice. The chapter also discussed doing research *with* people, not on them or to them, in keeping with the values of health promotion discussed throughout this book. The chapter provided discussion about participatory, creative methods of research as well as other methods which privilege people's voices and experiences such as qualitative approaches to research, discussing the ways in which these methods sit with the core values of the discipline. Attention was paid to power dynamic in the research process, as well as more specifically within research relationships and reflections on how to minimise these were also provided. Two case studies provided detail about anti-mainstream approaches, working with Indigenous ethics and using feminist principles in attempts to effect social change. This chapter informs the reader about how to do health promotion research in more ethical ways, irrespective of method, topic or indeed context.

Key points

- Health promotion research projects are diverse in methods, scope and focus, therefore this type of work constantly raises ethical challenges for researchers engaged in them. These challenges and appropriate responses are discussed in the literature in depth, and there are many guidelines for researchers to consult.
- Health promotion research should use traditional ethical guidelines but given that these have been criticised by many researchers, applying situated and negotiated ethics in each study is important to ensure that ethical challenges are managed well.
- Health promotion researchers should always consider contextual factors in relation to each study, and negotiate ethical parameters and issues with all involved, particularly participants, an on-going manner throughout the study.

Further reading

Kara, H. (2018) *Research Ethics in the Real World. Euro-Western and Indigenous Perspectives*. Bristol, Policy Press.
This book discusses research ethics in social, professional, institutional and political contexts. Kara compares Euro-western research traditions with those of indigenous community practices to show the reader the need for adapting ethical principles and practice in relation to context.
Potvin, L. & Didier, J. (2022 & 2023) *Global Handbook of Health Promotion Research, Volumes 1, 2 & 3*. New York, Springer.
The Global Handbook of Health Promotion Research consists of three distinct volumes, volume 1 is called mapping health promotion research, volume 2, is on framing health promotion research and volume 3 is about doing health promotion research. All three volumes contain edited book chapters from across the global discussing research in health promotion and how it is conducted. Reflection on challenges for health promotion research now and for the future are weaved throughout including those related to ethical research practice.
Warwick-Booth, L., Bagnall, AMB. & Coan, S. (2021) *Creating Participatory Research. Principles, Practice and Reality*. Bristol, Policy Press.
This book provides details about participatory research, and how participatory methods can be implemented in practice in an accessible and pragmatic manner, with a chapter focussing specifically on the ethics of doing this type of work (see Chapter 4). The ethics of doing participatory research, the principles beyond traditional guidance, examples of ethical practice, and a detailed case study, all encourage reader reflection. The book has an accompanying companion website, with further material about participatory research ethics available online.

References

Abma, T., Breed, M., Lips, S. and Schrijver, J. (2022) Whose voice is it really? Ethics of photovoice with children in health promotion. *International Journal of Qualitative Methods*, 21, 1–10.

Adekoya, A.A. and Guse, L. (2020) Walking interviews and wandering behavior: Ethical insights and methodological outcomes while exploring the perspectives of older adults living with dementia. *International Journal of Qualitative Methods*, 19, 1–6.

Al Tajir, G.K. (2018) Ethical treatment of participants in public health research. *Journal Public Health and Emergency*, 2, 2.

Armstrong, A., Aznarez, M., Banks, S., Henfrey, T. and Moore, H. et al. (2011) *Community-based Participatory Research: Ethical Challenges*, Durham, Durham University Centre for Social Justice and Community Action.

Banks, S., Armstrong, A., Carter, K., Graham, H., Hayward, P., Henry, A., Holland, T., Holmes, C., Lee, A., McNulty, A., Moore, N., Nayling, N., Stokoe, A. and Strachan, A. (2013) Everyday ethics in community-based participatory research. *Contemporary Social Science*, 8 (3), 263–277.

Black, G.F., Davies, A., Iskander, D. and Chambers, M. (2018) Reflection on the ethics of participatory visual methods to engage communities in global health research. *Global Bioethics*, 29 (1), 22–38.

Centre for Social Justice and Community Action (2012) *Community-based participatory research A guide to ethical principles and practice*. Centre for Social Justice and Community Action, Durham University National Co-ordinating Centre for Public Engagement.

Cornwall, A. and Jewkes, R. (1995) What is participatory research? *Social Science and Medicine*, 41 (12), 1667–1676.

Delderfield, R. (2018) When the researcher is a 'wounded storyteller': Exploring emotional labour and personal impact in research. The personal in the professional. *Self & Society*, 46 (2), 34–38.

Facca, D., Smith, M.J., Shelley, J., Lizotte, D. and Donelle, L.. (2020) Exploring the ethical issues in research using digital data collection strategies with minors: A scoping review. *PLoS One*. https://doi.org/10.1371/journal.pone.0237875

Flicker, S., Guta, A., Larkin, J., Flynn, S., Fridkin, A. and Travers, R. et al. (2010) Survey design from the ground up: Collaboratively creating the Toronto teen survey. *Health Promotion Practice*, 11 (1), 112–122.

Fogel, D.B. (2018) Factors associated with clinical trials that fail and opportunities for improving the likelihood of success: A review. *Contemporary Clinical Trials Communications*, 11, 156–164.

Garcia, R., Melgar, P. and Sorde, T.. (2013) In conversation with Cortes, L., Santiago, C. and Santiago, S. (Eds.), *Indigenous Pathways into Social Research: Voices of a New Generation*, pp. 367–380. California, Left Coast Press.

Gubrium, A.C., Hill, A.L. and Flicker, S. (2014) A situated practice of ethics for participatory visual and digital methods in public health research and practice: A focus on digital storytelling. *American Journal of Public Health*, 104 (9), 1606–1614.

Hall, A.C. (2019) Evaluations that fail: Nasty emails, small samples and tenuous futures. *Evidence & Policy*, 15 (1), 161–171.

IHPE (Institute of Health Promotion and Education) (2022) *IHPE Position Statement: Ethics and Health Promotion.* Retrieved from https://ihpe.org.uk/resources/position-papers/

Kara, H. (2017) *Academic taboos #1: what cannot be said.* Retrieved from https://helenkara.com/tag/ethics/

Kara, H. (2018) *Research Ethics in the Real World. Euro-Western and Indigenous Perspectives.* Bristol, Policy Press.

Kara, H. (2020) *Creative Research Methods. A Practical Guide.* 2nd Edn. Bristol, Policy Press.

Kawulich, B. and Ogletree, T.. (2012) Ethics in community research: Reflections from ethnographic research with first nations people in the US in Goodson, L. and Phillimore, J. (Eds.), *Community Research for Participation. From Theory to Method*, pp. 201–214. Bristol, Policy Press.

Kindon, S. (2003) Participatory video in geographic research: A feminist practice of looking? *Area*, 35 (2), 142–153.

Klinger, C., Barrett, D.H., Ondrusek, N., Johnsons, B.R. Jr., Saxena, A. and Reis, A.A. (2020) Beyond research ethics: Novel approaches of 3 major public health Institutions to provide ethics input on public health practice activities. *Journal of Public Health Management and Practice*, 26 (2), E12–E22. https://doi.org/10.1097/PHH.0000000000000734

Lavorgna, A. and Sugiura, L. (2020) Direct contacts with potential interviewees when carrying out online ethnography on controversial and polarized topics: A loophole in ethics guidelines. *International Journal of Social Research Methodology*, 25 (1). https://doi.org/10.1080/13645579.2020.1855719

London, A.J., Borasky, D.A. Jr. and Bhan, A. (2012) Improving ethical review of research involving incentives for health promotion. *PLOS Medicine*, 9 (3), e1001193.

Long, J.W., Ballard, H.L., Fisher, L. and Belskey, J.M. (2016) Questions that won't go away in participatory research. *Society and Natural Resources*, 29, 250–263.

Milgram, S. (1963) Behavioral study of obedience. *Journal of Abnormal and Social Psychology*, 67, 371–378.

Nind, M. (2017) The practical wisdom of inclusive research. *Qualitative Research*, 17 (3), 278–288.

Pause, C. (2017) Borderline: The ethics of fat stigma in public health. *Journal of Law, Medicine and Ethics*, 45, 510–517.

Rix, E., Wilson, S., Sheehan, N. and Tujague, N. (2018) Indigenist and decolonizing research methodology. In: Liamputtong, P. (Ed.), *Handbook of Research Methods in Health Social Sciences.* Singapore, Springer.

Samuel, G., Ballard, L.M., Carley, H. and Lucaseen, A.M.. (2022) Ethical preparedness in health research and care: The role of behavioural approaches. *BMC Medical Ethics*, 23, 115. https://doi.org/10.1186/s12910-022-00853-1

Shallwani, S. and Mohammed, S. (2007) *Community-based participatory research. A training manual for community-based researchers.* Retrieved from https://www.livingknowledge.org/fileadmin/Dateien-Living-Knowledge/Dokumente_Dateien/Toolbox/LK_A_Training_manual.pdf

Shaw, J. (2016) Emergent ethics in participatory video: Negotiating the inherent tensions as group processes evolve in Special Section: Critiquing participatory video: Experiences from around the world. *Area*, 48 (4), 419–426.

Shaw, J. (2021) Extended participatory video processes. In: Burns, D., Howard, J. and Ospina, S. (Eds.), *The SAGE Handbook of Participatory Research and Enquiry*. London, Sage Publishing.

Sime, D. (2008) Ethical and methodological issues in engaging young people in poverty with participatory methods. *Children's Geographies*, 6 (1), 63–78.

Smith, C. (2013) Becoming a Kaupapa Maori researcher. In: Mertens, D., Cram, F. and Chilisia, B. (Eds.), *Indigenous Pathways into Social Research: Voices of a New Generation*, pp. 89–99. California, Left Coast Press.

Staley, K. and Elliot, J. (2017) Public involvement could usefully inform ethical review, but rarely does: What are the implications *Research Involvement and Engagement*, 3, 30. https://doi.org/10.1186/s40900-017-0080-0

Tamariz, L., Palacio, A., Robert, M. and Marcus, E.N. (2013) Improving the informed consent process for research subjects with low literacy: A systematic review. *Journal of General Internal Medicine*, 28 (1), 121–126.

Terry, L. (2016) *Refreshing Perspectives. Exploring the Application of Peer Research with Populations Facing Severe and Multiple Disadvantage*. London, Revolving Doors Agency & Lankelly Chase.

Warwick-Booth, L., Bagnall, A.M. and Coan, S. (2021) *Creating Participatory Research. Principles, Practice and Reality*. Bristol, Policy Press.

Warwick-Booth, L. and Coan, S. (2022) *Using qualitative online methods to evaluate community responses to Covid19 SAGE Research Methods: Doing research online*. Retrieved from https://methods.sagepub.com/

Warwick-Booth, L., Cross, R. and Coan, S. (2023) The practices of feminist stakeholders supporting social change and health improvement for women experiencing domestic abuse in England. In: Jourdon, D. & Potvin, L. (Eds.), *Global Handbook on Health Promotion Research. Doing Health Promotion Research*, Volume 3. New York, Springer.

Woodall, J. (2010) *Control and choice in three category-C English prisons: Implications for the concept and practice of the health promoting prison*, PhD Thesis, Leeds Beckett University.

Woodall, J., Cross, R., Kinsella, K. and Bunyon, A.M. (2018a) Using peer research processes to understand strategies to support those with severe, multiple and complex health needs. *Health Education Journal*, 78 (2), 176–188.

Woodall, J., Kinsella, K., Cross, R. and Bunyon, A.M. and inspiring change Manchester's Peer researchers. (2016) *Service Users Experiences of Inspiring Change Manchester* Leeds. Leeds Beckett University.

Woodall, J., Warwick-Booth, L., South, J. and Cross, R. (2018b) What makes health promotion research distinct? *Scandinavian Journal of Public Health*, 46 (Suppl. 20), 118–122.

6   Ethics, evaluation and evidence-based practice

Introduction

This chapter introduces the ethical implications with respect to evaluation, evidence and evidence-based practice in health promotion. Evaluation is a critical component of the health promotion planning process – a cyclical approach to identifying aims, interventions and evaluating success to refine delivery. Evaluation derives evidence and both feed into evidence-based practice which is an important concept in delivering high-quality, effective interventions and programmes. By the end of this chapter, the reader should be able to:

- Understand the imperative to evaluate health promotion activity as part of the planning process, but recognise that this can come with ethical tensions;
- Appreciate the impact of evaluation activity on individuals and organisations and how this can cause anxiety if undertaken poorly;
- Recognise the range of possible indicators to determine success in health promotion activities and how these indicators may require ethical consideration;
- Acknowledge the ethics concerning evidence-based decision-making and the types and quality of evidence to make decisions.

The ethical imperative to evaluate

Evaluation is a key competency for health promotion practitioners and acknowledged as being essential to the development of evidence and subsequently the discipline and practice (Barry et al., 2009; Woodall and Cross, 2021). A credible discipline requires an evidence base with which practitioners and decision makers can base their practice decisions on (Deehan and Wylie, 2010). There are strong ethical perspectives linked to robust evaluation of health promotion activity and, as noted earlier in the book (see Chapter 4), it is critical that health promotion

DOI: 10.4324/9781003308317-6

interventions do not derive unintended outcomes and unhelpful consequences. Evaluation is central in being able to identify what works (and why it works); and to identify any unintended side effects caused by health promotion activities. Theoretically then, evaluation would enable evidence to be generated to highlight good practice and to show practices that cause harm and therefore not to be replicated elsewhere.

Some of the reasons why evaluation is crucial include:

- To improve the design or performance of a project, policy, service, etc.;
- To make choices between health promotion activities;
- To aid decisions about which activities should be funded and which have greatest impact;
- To learn how a project might be repeated and sustained elsewhere;
- For accountability – to check it is going to plan;
- To find out if a project provides value for money;
- To test new and innovative ideas (Wright, 1999).

Evaluation is a critical element of health promotion practice and in generating an evidence base to aid future practice. It is, of course, intimately intertwined with the health promotion planning process and sets out to achieve laudable goals as outlined in the list above. With this in mind, the reader can be forgiven in wondering why ethics is discussed vis-à-vis evaluation and evidence. However, as will be demonstrated the ethical challenges posed by evaluation are numerous.

Ethics and evaluation: some dilemmas

Given the opening section of the chapter has made a strong case for evaluation activity in health promotion, there are some situations where evaluation is not an ethical activity. Green and South (2006) consider occasions when evaluation would not be appropriate. These scenarios include:

- Evaluation would not represent an ethical use of resources because it would divert time, staff and funds from essential activities;
- Evaluation would place an unacceptable burden on practitioners and other stakeholders;
- Communities or organisations have been overresearched and do not want to be evaluated;
- Evaluation would be too intrusive or risk generating conflict in areas of work where there are major social, political or cultural tensions;
- It is not possible to carry out an evaluation of sufficient depth and quality to aid decision-making;
- Evaluators would be compromised and would not be free to report findings accurately.

Reflection on Practice 6.1

Try to consider further ethical considerations in relation to appointing appropriate evaluators. What further ethical tensions could arise from conducting internal evaluations and when might such an approach be entirely reasonable and pragmatic?

Whilst most people agree on the importance of evaluation, it is often done poorly or even omitted (Hubley et al., 2021). One particular issue is whether an organisation can evaluate themselves, or if an external organisation is required to provide objective scrutiny (see Reflection on Practice 6.1). The literature suggests an increasing rise in the amount of 'in-house' evaluation conducted by individuals on their own organisation (Pattyn and Brans, 2013). The reasons for this could be manifold but might include anxieties about being evaluated by third parties (discussed later) or the financial implications of hiring an external evaluator or academic researcher. A general guideline is that between 5% and 10% of a programme budget should be allocated to evaluation, but in reality this is rarely the case.

Internal evaluators could become objectively compromised by the politics of their organisation and may feel some pressure to report positive outcomes. This creates some concerns about impartiality and whether the findings of an internal evaluator are robust or could stand up to outside scrutiny (Pattyn and Brans, 2013). On the other hand, being an 'insider' can illuminate rich and detailed information that could be difficult to access by externally appointed evaluation teams. Whilst not always the case, there could be issues in relation to skills and expertise in relation to evaluation design that may be better procured through outsourcing. This might be the case where health promotion interventions are more complex or if a particular methodological approach is required (e.g. a cost-effectiveness study which relies on highly technical skill sets). There are a range of practitioner barriers to evaluation which have been highlighted by Wright (1999). These include:

- Concerns about competence:
  - *'I am not an academic'*
  - *'I don't know the language'*
  - *'I don't know statistics'*
- Concerns about quality:
  - *'What is good enough research'*
  - *'What level should I be working at'*

- Concerns about time and resources:
  - *'How can I fit this in'*
  - *'I don't have time'*
  - *'I have to get on with doing health promotion'*
- Concerns and dissemination and implementation:
  - *'If I do this research, will any care'*
  - *'I can't produce anything worth publishing'*
  - *'Will the research be useful'*

Anxiety and the evaluation process is a further ethical conundrum. People do not generally like their projects being evaluated (Hall, 2019). Being scrutinised by others on your practice or ways of working can be inherently threatening and disconcerting and in some cases can cause excessive evaluation anxiety (XEA) where practitioners being evaluated block evaluators from accessing information and/or are unwilling to co-operate with the evaluation process (Bechar and Mero-Jaffe, 2014). Apprehension and resistance to evaluation is a common phenomenon in general (Moretti, 2021) and no doubt applies in health promotion evaluations also (see Reflection on Practice 6.2). Evaluators must reduce anxieties and concerns as it is apparent that evaluation activity can stir up significant emotions concerning loss of employment, reputational damage, fear of retribution, and fear of feeling undermined or undervalued (Moretti, 2021).

One promising development in the public health field, is the use of embedded researchers (ERs) – these individuals sit both objectively and subjectively in organisations and are often a middle ground between in-house evaluation and external scrutiny. ERs are becoming more commonplace with a range of examples being published in public health (Homer et al., 2022; Potts et al., 2022). Similar to other methodological strategies, ER has been defined in various ways by various commentators. Most definitions, however, acknowledge that ERs are individuals who are often university based and employed to undertake explicit research roles within host organisations (McGinity and Salokangas, 2014; Vindrola-Padros et al., 2017), such as local authority public

---

Reflection on Practice 6.2

Evidence suggests that evaluations can cause a range of adverse concerns, anxieties and fears in people – ethically this is unacceptable and should be eradicated. What steps and measures should be considered when undertaking an evaluation to reduce these impacts? You may wish to refer to Chapter 5 to help with this.

health departments or voluntary or community sector organisations. ERs have gained popularity for a myriad of reasons. Effective knowledge exchange is cited as a primary benefit as ERs are often able to align research rigour, situational context and independence with practical application for policy and practice in the host organisation (Wolfenden et al., 2017). There is a challenge though for ERs to undertake their work expediently – and perhaps in a rushed way – in order to meet the needs of decision makers who require evidence to inform policy in an almost instantaneous fashion. This perhaps reiterates the cultural tensions that ERs can face. Indeed, it is often the case that policy decisions can frequently be underpinned by political timeliness (based on perceived short-term opportunities and political preferences), rather than credible research evidence (van de Goor et al., 2017). Linked to this, is that ERs within host organisation are often *the* only resource for undertaking research – this can be frustrating and can sometimes lead to host organisations having unrealistic expectations of what an ER may be able to achieve in their practice (Wye et al., 2019).

What counts as success in evaluation and has change *really* occurred?

There is an array of ways in which success in health promoting interventions can be measured and indeed, given the complexity of many programmes, having a range of measurement tools is advantageous to capture the outcomes that may be possible. Box 6.1 shows some of the

---

Box 6.1   Measuring success in health promotion – some common measures and some ethical challenges

- *Changes in health outcomes (e.g. increased life expectancy, reduced morbidity and increased quality of life)*
  A health promotion intervention, which is able to demonstrate clearly that it is able to deliver positive changes in health outcomes, is highly desirable. However, showing that a programme or policy or activity can, say, increase someone's life expectancy is very difficult to say. This is because there are a whole range of other factors (outside of the intervention) that may be influencing that. It would also require an evaluation that could track outcomes over a long period of time. In most cases, it is impossible for small-scale health promotion interventions to make legitimate claims about their impact on life expectancy. Nonetheless, it may be feasible to look at proxy measures that might be less complex to measure such as improved quality of life in the short term.

- *Behaviour change (e.g. increased physical activity, reduced alcohol usage and dietary change)*
  These types of measurements are very common in health promotion evaluation and relatively easy to administer and design. Change can be demonstrated over a relatively short period of time which can indicate the success, or not, of an intervention which intends to modify behaviour. There are broader ethical critiques of these programmes and indeed the evaluation of them – some might suggest that the behaviours themselves are manifestation of deeper issues (such as poverty, education, etc.) that should be tackled and evaluated for their success. Political cycles and electoral timelines can mean that these measures can be very popular to show progress made around key health objectives and the findings from such evaluations can be easier to understand for people and the media (e.g. '25% of residents now more physically active than last year' or 'smoking rates down by half').

- *Increased knowledge and awareness (e.g. more knowledgeable about how to reduce the transmission of communicable disease)*
  Knowledge and attitudes can be measured using recognised scales and research tools. Measuring knowledge can be done easily and are good indicators for measuring short-term impact. That said, change in knowledge or attitude does not necessarily imply changing behaviour.

- *Skills acquisition (e.g. being able to cook healthy food)*
  For some programmes, this is a useful indicator of success. Nonetheless, it is important to consider not only skill acquisition but also whether the skill is being used in day-to-day life.

- *Increased empowerment*
  Several health promotion initiatives aim to empower individuals and communities, but few are able to evaluate success effectively. The reasons for this are complex but include the lack of an agreed definition of empowerment which makes comparing the effectiveness of initiatives troublesome. One initiative's version and conceptualisation of empowerment could be very different to another's. Individual notions of empowerment tend to be easier to measure (self-esteem, control, etc.), but empowerment is far wider than this.

common indicators of success used in health promotion, but with the addition of ethical critique surrounding their usage.

Most evaluations comprised two components. First, the assessment of outcomes – that is the changes that result from an intervention. The intervention could be a programme or a policy, for example, and the purpose is to determine what, if anything, has changed as a result of that intervention. In contrast, the assessment of process is looking at the mechanisms operating within interventions and the influence of contextual factors (South and Woodall, 2012).

In relation to establishing outcomes from an intervention – one ethical question is whether the outcomes are *really* a result of the health promotion activity and whether we can confidently attribute cause and effect. One way to increase the confidence that changed has occurred through a health promotion intervention, and not by chance or fluke, is to utilise randomised control trials (RCTs) which can provide greater certainty than other designs. The RCT is an experimental process in which people or communities are randomly selected to one of two groups: one (the experimental group) receiving the intervention that is being tested and the other (the comparison group or control) receiving either an alternative or nothing at all. The two groups are then followed up to see if there are any differences between them. This will demonstrate the effectiveness of the intervention and whether it has positive or negative impacts (see an example in Case Study 6.1).

Case Study 6.1   Evaluation of the impact of a school gardening intervention on children's fruit and vegetable intake: a randomised controlled trial

The RCT is often criticised for being incompatible with the values and philosophy of health promotion, but the RCT has been used to good effect in some cases. Christian et al. (2014) demonstrated, using a cluster randomisation of schools, the effectiveness of a school gardening programme on children's fruit and vegetable intake. The study evaluated the impact of a Royal Horticultural Society (RHS)-led intervention against a less involved teacher-led intervention.

Ten schools in London were randomly allocated to receive the RHS-led intervention and 13 schools were allocated to receive the teacher-led intervention. The results have found very little evidence to support the claims that school gardening alone can improve children's daily fruit and vegetable intake. Nonetheless, when a gardening intervention is implemented at a high level within the school, it may improve children's daily fruit and vegetable intake by a portion.

Within health promotion, there are some concerns about the ethics of the RCT and its applicability. Green et al. (2019) have summarised these as follows:

- Inability to cope with the complexity of health promotion programmes;
- RCTs do not pay sufficient attention to process and the quality of interventions;
- Practical difficulties in relation to randomisation;
- Contamination of control or reference groups;
- Are ideologically incompatible with health promotion in relation to:
  - commitment to 'active' individual and community participation in the research process;
  - contributing to its empowering and 'emancipatory' role;
  - the use of research as a tool for achieving political and social changes.

Health promotion as a practice then is in a challenging position. There are legitimate calls for a stronger evidence base and a firmer understanding of what works. However, using some evaluation designs (i.e. RCTs) can be ethically and practically challenging and contradictory to the underpinning values of health promotion.

Ethical challenges to evidence-based health promotion

Undertaking health promotion activity using evidence-based principles is a very positive approach as it provides some assurances that interventions are more likely to succeed based on sound empirical understanding (Woodall and Rowlands, 2020). Perkins et al. (1999), however, provide some challenge to this. First, how much evidence is required before action can be taken and what level of uncertainty within the evidence can be tolerated? This is a crucial point, as evidence on many topics is not always completely conclusive and can often be contradictory. Would one, well designed and robust study be enough to base a decision? Or would further research be needed to verify these results? (Woodall and Cross, 2021).

Second, the tension between different types of knowledge and what types of evidence decision makers may privilege – either implicitly or explicitly. In health disciplines and in medical sciences, there are some very well-established views on what constitutes evidence. These views often describe different types of evidence and categorises them as higher quality and lower quality. This is often seen as a hierarchy with 'gold standard' research designs producing more reliable or effective evidence than others (see Box 6.2). Early ideas of the hierarchy were initially led

Box 6.2 The evidence hierarchy

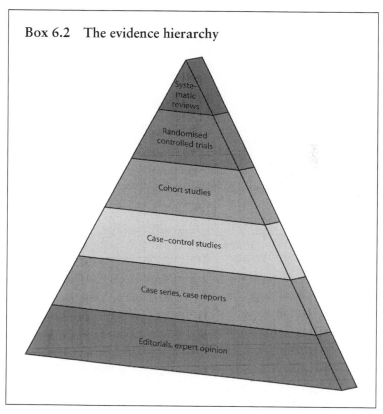

Systematic reviews

Randomised controlled trials

Cohort studies

Case–control studies

Case series, case reports

Editorials, expert opinion

by the Canadian Task Force on the Periodic Health Examination to help decide on priorities when searching for studies to answer clinical questions (Petticrew and Roberts, 2003) and was only later considered for its implications for public health and health promotion evidence.

Using a range of evidence within health promotion in order to inform policy and practice decisions is now understood and this has meant abandoning hierarchies of evidence towards typologies of evidence (Woodall and Rowlands, 2020), but there remains still some reluctance to engage with less traditional evidence sources. Case Study 6.2 shows how different forms of evidence can be used together to aid decision-making processes but perhaps also shows the ethical tensions between how much 'trust' commissioners place in particular forms of data.

Perkins et al. (1999) also outline the tension between inspiration and evidence, highlighting the extent to which tried and tested methods are used – which may have a firm evidence base – in contrast to

Case Study 6.2   Age-friendly environment and community-based social innovation in Japan: a mixed-method study

Abstract

Background and objectives

Whilst governments are building age-friendly environments, community-based social innovation (CBSI) provides opportunities for older community residents to interact. Common CBSIs in Japan are in the form of group exercise activities or social–cultural activities, such as reading, writing, poetry, chorus, calligraphy, card game, knitting, planting trees and cooking. In this study, an age-friendly environment in Japan was assessed quantitatively and qualitatively through the perceptions of community residents and their interaction with the environment.

Research design and methods

A cross-sectional survey of 243 participants and multiple in-depth interviews were carried out. A quantitative study applied the World Health Organisation (WHO) framework of 20 age-friendly environmental factors with analysis applying a structural equation model. A qualitative study applied focus group meetings and in-depth interviews to conduct a thematic analysis of Japanese community residents' activities according to the WHO scope of CBSI for healthy aging.

Results

This age-friendly environment in Japan has provided pathways for the older people to sustain their social network, which promotes civic participation and engagement in peer group activities leading to active aging. CBSIs are the factors that lead to an age-friendly environment resulting in a sustainable quality of life.

Discussion and implications

It is important to sustain CBSIs in the era of coronavirus disease 2019 pandemic as those are the paths leading to healthy aging communities and quality of older residents' life. The lessons learned about how physical environment and social participation result in healthy, active quality of life for older adults in Japan may be applicable to other contexts around the world.

Source: Aung et al. (2021)

Reflection on Practice 6.3

What would you do if there was insufficient, high-quality, evidence to make a useful decision on the delivery of an intervention? How would you be confident that the decision you were making had the highest likelihood to succeed despite a lack of evidence?

---

innovative and creative solutions to problems. As shown in Reflection on Practice 6.3, it may be that a wedded fixation with evidence-based decision-making has its limitations and that it may be prudent to allow some innovative practice to be conducted alongside careful evaluation of the delivery (Woodall and Cross, 2021).

Access to evidence: an ethical concern?

Linked to the broader ethical debates surrounding evidence-based health promotion is the challenge of accessing evidence and research that has been published. Evidence that underpins decision-making is likely, although not exclusively, to be obtained via academic sources such as journal articles and research literature. This is because these sources are often regarded as being more robust, credible and reviewed by experts in the field (known as peer review). According to Woodall and Cross (2021), access to journal articles has been traditionally done in three ways:

1 Access via the journal website;
2 Accessing a physical copy via a library;
3 Accessing the journal via an academic database.

Practitioners can struggle to access literature as many journals are subscription based and cost money to be affiliated with. This is known to cause some challenges in accessing contemporary and up to date sources (Homer et al., 2022) – this issue may be intensified in lower and middle-income countries where resource allocation may be particularly challenging. Open access (OA) publications, however, are free and unrestricted online research journals that allow access to research evidence. They ensure that research is easily accessible to practitioners, policy makers and researchers without a cost. Traditional publishing models mean that journals usually have a subscription cost which means that research can be inaccessible to many. Some excellent examples of OA journals which frequently feature health promotion studies include BMJ Open, BMC Public Health and Global Health (PLOS ONE).

Reflection on Practice 6.4

Take a topic that you are passionate about and identify key research studies in this field. Make a note about which studies might
be inaccessible to you and consider how you might be able to
overcome this. Also, try to find 'grey' unpublished literature on
your topic. How would you go about finding this? How confident
would you be in using the findings or conclusions to inform your
practice?

A further ethical issue is where results of evaluation or research studies are not published or withheld which can mean that negative results
of intervention evaluations are underreported or not reported at all. This
means that gathering a 'full picture' of the evidence can be difficult given
that these studies may be held in local organisations and difficult to access
via traditional search methods. Searching for this 'grey literature' is crucial, as it can provide contextual information on how, why and for whom
interventions are effective (Adams et al., 2016). The drawback, however,
is that grey literature has not gone through rigorous peer review as would
be expected in many journals. Training practitioners and researchers in
accessing grey literature is not always a priority and instead more ortho-
dox methods of retrieving studies are used in training and education contexts. Perhaps as technology continues to develop at a rapid pace and
the blurring between published and non-published literature becomes ever
more apparent through the internet, more attention will be paid to accessing grey literature to inform evidence-based practice. An opportunity to
think further about this is featured in Reflection on Practice 6.4.

Summary

This chapter has sought to demonstrate some of the ethical tensions
that can occur when evaluating and assessing evidence in health promotion. The chapter established that evaluation is a crucial component
to developing evidence-based practice, but highlighted ethical tensions
concerning the evaluation process. This includes anxiety caused through
evaluation processes and the dilemma between in-house and external
scrutiny when evaluation interventions. The measures adopted to evaluating success in health promotion interventions were also discussed with
some ethical caveats surrounding the use of long-term outcomes, such
as life expectancy, as a useful measure for some health promotion programmes. The application of RCTs in health promotion evaluation was

also highlighted and whilst this design can be highly robust and valid, there are ethical concerns about its application in complex community programmes. That said, several successful RCTs have been delivered in health promotion and revealed important results. Finally, accessing evidence as an ethical concern was highlighted and how this can be overcome through developments in open access publishing.

Key points

- Evaluation is critical to health promotion planning and forms a key part in evidence-based decision-making and practice.
- There are several ethical tensions concerning evaluation practices in health promotion. For instance, whether 'in-house' evaluation offers the objectivity required for credible conclusions on practice.
- Indicators that measure the success of health promotion interventions must be carefully considered. Increasing an individual or a community's knowledge on a given health issue may not lead to any behavioural outcomes.
- The design chosen to evaluate health promotion interventions requires ethical scrutiny. The RCT is a good example of a research design that may not always be suited to complex health interventions.
- Accessing good-quality evidence can be difficult and practitioners can sometimes be 'blocked' from retrieving the best studies to inform their decision-making and practices.

Further reading

Green J and South J. (2006) *Evaluation*. Maidenhead, Open University Press.
Hubley, J., Copeman, J. and Woodall, J. (2021) *Practical Health Promotion*. Cambridge, Polity Press.
Woodall, J. and Cross, R. (2021) *Essentials of Health Promotion*. London, Sage.

References

Adams, J., Hillier-Brown, F.C., Moore, H.J., Lake, A.A., Araujo-Soares, V., White, M. and Summerbell, C. (2016) Searching and synthesising 'grey literature' and 'grey information' in public health: Critical reflections on three case studies. *Systematic Reviews*, 5, 164.
Aung, M.N., Koyanagi, Y., Ueno, S., Tiraphat, S. and Yuasa, M. (2021) Age-friendly environment and community-based social innovation in Japan: A mixed-method study. *The Gerontologist*, 62, 89–99.
Barry, M.M., Allegrante, J.P., Lamarre, M.-C., Auld, M.E. and Taub, A. (2009) The Galway Consensus Conference: International collaboration on the development of core competencies for health promotion and health education. *Global Health Promotion*, 16, 5–11.

112 *Ethics, evaluation and evidence-based practice*

Bechar, S. and Mero-Jaffe, I. (2014) Who is afraid of evaluation? Ethics in evaluation research as a way to cope with excessive evaluation anxiety: Insights from a case study. *American Journal of Evaluation*, 35, 364–376.

Christian, M.S., Evans, C.E.L., Nykjaer, C., Hancock, N. and Cade, J.E. (2014) Evaluation of the impact of a school gardening intervention on children's fruit and vegetable intake: A randomised controlled trial. *International Journal of Behavioral Nutrition and Physical Activity*, 11, 99.

Deehan, A. and Wylie, A. (2010) Health promotion: The challenges, the questions of definition, discipline status and evidence base. In: Wylie, A., Holt, T. and Howe, A. (Eds.), *Health Promotion in Medical Education: from Rhetoric to Action*. Oxford, Radcliffe Publishing.

Green, J., Cross, R., Woodall, J. and Tones, K. (2019) *Health Promotion. Planning and Strategies*. London, Sage.

Green, J. and South, J. (2006) *Evaluation*. Maidenhead, Open University Press.

Hall, A.C. (2019) Evaluations that fail: Nasty emails, small samples and tenuous futures. *Evidence & Policy: A Journal of Research, Debate and Practice*, 15, 161–172.

Homer, C., Woodall, J., Freeman, C., South, J., Cooke, J., Holliday, J., Hartley, A. and Mullen, S. (2022) Changing the culture: A qualitative study exploring research capacity in local government. *BMC Public Health*, 22, 1–10.

Hubley, J., Copeman, J. and Woodall, J. (2021) *Practical Health Promotion*. Cambridge, Polity Press.

McGinity, R. and Salokangas, M. (2014) Introduction: 'Embedded research' as an approach into academia for emerging researchers. *Management in Education*, 28, 3–5.

Moretti, E. (2021) Navigating the awkward, challenging social context of evaluation. *Evaluation Journal of Australasia*, 21, 163–176.

Pattyn, V. and Brans, M. (2013) Outsource versus in-house? An identification of organizational conditions influencing the choice for internal or external evaluators. *Canadian Journal of Program Evaluation*, 28.

Perkins, S., Simnett, I. and Wright, L. (1999) Creative tensions in evidence-based practice. In: Perkins, E.R., Simnett, I. and Wright, L. (Eds.), *Evidence Based Health Promotion*. Chichester, John Wiley & Sons.

Petticrew, M. and Roberts, H. (2003) Evidence, hierarchies, and typologies: Horses for courses. *Journal of Epidemiology and Community Health*, 57, 527–529.

Potts, A.J., Nobles, J., Shearn, K., Danks, K. and Frith, G. (2022) Embedded researchers as part of a whole systems approach to physical activity: Reflections and recommendations. *Systems*, 10, 69.

South, J. and Woodall, J. (2012) Planning and evaluating health promotion in settings. In: Scriven, A. and Hodgins, M. (Eds.), *Health Promotion Settings: Principles and Practice*. London, Sage.

van de Goor, I., Hämäläinen, R.-M., Syed, A., Juel Lau, C., Sandu, P., Spitters, H., Eklund Karlsson, L., Dulf, D., Valente, A., Castellani, T. and Aro, A.R. (2017) Determinants of evidence use in public health policy making: Results from a study across six EU countries. *Health Policy*, 121, 273–281.

Vindrola-Padros, C., Pape, T., Utley, M. and Fulop, N.J. (2017) The role of embedded research in quality improvement: A narrative review. *BMJ Quality & Safety*, 26, 70–80.

Wolfenden, L., Yoong, S.L., Williams, C.M., Grimshaw, J., Durrheim, D.N., Gillham, K. and Wiggers, J. (2017) Embedding researchers in health service organizations improves research translation and health service performance: The Australian Hunter New England Population Health example. *Journal of Clinical Epidemiology*, 85, 3–11.

Woodall, J. and Cross, R. (2021) *Essentials of Health Promotion*. London, Sage.

Woodall, J. and Rowlands, S. (2020) Professional practice. In: Cross, R., Foster, S., O'neil, I., Rowlands, S., Woodall, J. and Warwick-Booth, L. (Eds.), *Health Promotion: Global Principles and Practice*. London, CABI.

Wright, L. (1999) Doing things right. In: Perkins, E.R., Simnett, I. and Wright, L. (Eds.), *Evidence Based Health Promotion*. Chichester, John Wiley & Sons.

Wye, L., Cramer, H., Carey, J., Anthwal, R., Rooney, J., Robinson, R., Beckett, K., Farr, M., le May, A. and Baxter, H. (2019) Knowledge brokers or relationship brokers? The role of an embedded knowledge mobilisation team. *Evidence & Policy*, 15, 277–292.

7 Towards an ethical future in health promotion

Introduction

This chapter considers what an ethical future in health promotion might look like. It picks up on the main themes presented the previous six chapters and has two distinct halves. In the first half of the chapter we discuss codes of ethics in health promotion drawing on some existing frameworks and guidelines for health promotion practice. We reflect on how ethical values and principles underpin these and consider how they might be further developed for best practice. In doing so we pick up on the discussion about ethical frameworks that was introduced in Chapter 2. The latter half of this chapter covers issues of sustainability taking into account the sustainability of health promotion and sustainability in relation to planetary health, and what it means to work ethically in relation to these. We discuss the collective responsibility that those working in health promotion have to work in ethically sustainable ways to promote health and end by considering redistributive policy as a means to a more ethical future.

By the end of this chapter the reader should be able to:

- Appreciate how ethics and ethical considerations underpin several health promotion frameworks for practice;
- Understand issues of sustainability in relation to health promotion action and planetary health;
- Appreciate how ecological approaches are crucial to health promotion's contribution to tackling issues such as climate change;
- Understand how collective action is critical to tackling issues relating to social justice and planetary health.

Ethical codes of practice

Chapter 4 briefly introduced the idea of ethical codes of practice; in this chapter we will explore this idea in more depth. We begin by examining ethics in relation to several health promotion competency frameworks.

DOI: 10.4324/9781003308317-7

As defined by Woodall and Cross (2022, p. 219) a competency framework is 'a structure that sets out the individual competencies that are required from someone working in a specific profession, institution or organisation'. Without exception the competency frameworks for health promotion practice in existence have ethics at the core. Competency frameworks tend to set out the skills, abilities, values and knowledge that people working in health promotion will need which are all underpinned by an understanding of ethics that informs decisions and actions to promote health.

Country-specific frameworks

It is noteworthy that competency frameworks and codes of practice tend to have been developed in the global north in a minority of wealthier countries and in the past decade or so; however, we will spend some time considering these in relation to their ethical foundations. Starting with the UK, which is where we are writing from, we have seen a shift away from health promotion towards public health in more recent times. In 2009, the Society of Health Education and Promotion Specialists in Wales and the Shaping the Future Collaboration (led by the Royal Society of Public Health in partnership with the Faculty of Public Health, the UK Public Health Register and the Institute of Health Promotion and Education) collaborated on *A Framework for Ethical Health Promotion*. This framework includes consideration of the principles of health promotion practice but is not actually a code of conduct. Some of the areas this framework covers echo the content of Chapter 2 and are worth reiterating in Table 7.1.

In the absence of any specific health promotion code of conduct there is the *UK-wide Public Health Skills and Knowledge Framework* (PHSKF, 2016) which guides current health promotion and public health practice. It was first published in 2016 and then updated in 2019. Ethics are considered within this framework in terms of professional and ethical underpinnings and are specifically referenced as follows:

- 'promote ethical practice with an understanding of the ethical dilemmas that might be faced when promoting population health and reducing health inequalities;
- identify and apply ethical frameworks when faced with difficult decisions when promoting the public's health and reducing inequalities' (PHSKF, 2016, p. 9).

These are seen to underpin the functions and sub-functions detailed in the framework itself; however, as mentioned previously, this framework

Table 7.1 Ethical Health Promotion (SHEPS Cymru and Shaping the Future, 2009)

General Ethical Principles	• Do good (beneficence) • Avoid doing harm (non-maleficence) • Respect for autonomy • Justice
Ultimate Goals	Including: • Health as a basis human right • Holistic understanding of health • Equity in health • Empowerment
Ways of Working	Including: • Addressing the needs of disadvantaged and marginalised groups • Working participatively • Enabling individuals and communities to have control over their health, i.e. in ways which are empowering • Working in partnership with individuals, communities and sectors • Endeavouring to ensure that services have long-term positive effects • Encouraging social responsibility for health and individuals' responsibility for their own health • Attempting to counter discrimination • Promoting trust • A commitment to sustainable development and a socio-ecological model of health

was developed with reference to public health rather than health promotion (see Chapter 1 to revisit the distinctions between public health and health promotion as we see them).

The second edition of the Australian '*Foundation Competencies for Public Health Graduates in Australia*' (Somerset et al., 2016) builds on the first edition published in 2009 and also represents the core competencies required from health promotion practitioners. It explicitly states that 'an understanding of ethics is fundamental knowledge for all Public Health graduates' (p. 3). One of the units of competency under the 'Evidence-based Professional Population Health Practice' area of practice is to be able to 'describe core principles of just, ethical/legal public health practice' (p. 21). Ethics is also specifically mentioned in relation to ethical indigenous health practice but, in a document that is 46 pages long, the word 'ethics' only appears four times. The word 'ethical' appears 14 times in relation to ethical principles and ethical practice.

However, the functions, competencies and characteristics of the role are described as that of an 'ethical and judgment safe professional public health practitioner' (p. 35). It is assumed, of course, that the practitioner's underpinning values are concordant with, and support, ethical and judgements about safe practice.

One of the few countries to have a specific health promotion competency framework is Canada, in the form of the '*Pan-Canadian Health Promoter Competencies and Glossary*' which was published by Health Promotion Canada in 2015. The word 'ethical' appears twice in this; first with reference to the combinations of approaches that health promoters might use when it states that health promoters should 'champion ways of working based in evidence of effectiveness, theory and clear ethical principles' (p. 4) and then again under Leadership and Building Organizational Capacity where it is stated that the health promoter should be able to 'Manage self, others, information and resources in an ethical manner' (p. 10). The word 'ethics' does not appear at all in the 20-page document.

The Health Promotion Forum of New Zealand (2012) has published a set of competencies for health promotion that was most recently updated in 2022 – *Ngā Kaiakatanga Hauora mō Aotearoa: Health Promotion Competencies for Aotearoa New Zealand*. New Zealand has an existing code of ethics for public health, but the document references a 'yet to be developed' code of ethics for health promotion. Nevertheless, it is stated that 'a health promoter will demonstrate their commitment to ethical practice by acting according to the code of ethics for health promotion practice' (p. 10). Values and ethics underpin the nine competency clusters that appear in the competency framework which specifically reflect the traditional values of the indigenous people of New Zealand including the Māori and Pacific people and Pacific nations. This document emphasises that competencies should be context specific and details competencies that are specific to the Māori context. Arguably this is the most ethical approach to developing competency frameworks in health promotion since such an approach will take into account the socio-cultural context in which the health promoter is working in Take some time to carry out Reflection on Practice 7.1.

International frameworks

At the time of writing this chapter it was not possible to identify any specific health promotion competency frameworks from the global south; however, there has been a body of work in recent years by the International Union of Health Promotion and Education (IUHPE) that has attempted to produce an international set of health promotion competencies. The global health promotion community fed into the process of

---

Reflection on Practice 7.1

Having considered several country-specific competency frameworks take some time to reflect on what you consider to be the core competencies that a health promoter needs for practice. Where do you think ethics and ethical practice come into this process and how are they reflected in specific competencies? You might want to look at the following frameworks as you reflect on this:

Health Promotion Forum of New Zealand – *Ngā Kaiakatanga Hauora mō Aotearoa: Health Promotion Competencies for Aotearoa New Zealand* www.hauora.co.nz

Australian Health Promotion Association – *Core Competencies for Health Promotion Practitioners* www.healthpromotion. org.au

Health Promotion Canada – *Pan-Canadian Health Promoter Competencies and Glossary* www.healthpromotioncanada.ca

---

developing this set of competencies was led by Professor Margaret Barry and colleagues and took place over several years resulting in the *IUHPE Core Competencies and Professional Standards for Health Promotion* (IUHPE, 2016). There are nine competency domains as follows:

1 Enable change
2 Advocate for health
3 Mediate through partnership
4 Communication
5 Leadership
6 Assessment
7 Planning
8 Implementation, and
9 Evaluation and research

You will note that this list of competency domains reflects many of the things we have covered in this book. Two further domains underpin all of the nine domains – health promotion knowledge and ethical values, resulting in 11 domains in total. In the Framework's Handbook it is stated that 'ethical values are integral to the practice of health promotion and form the context within which all other competencies are practiced' (Dempsey et al., 2011, p. 7). The complexity of health promotion practice is reflected in the number of competency statements in this framework – there are 68 in total (Bull et al., 2012; Van Den Broucke, 2021). Similarly to the country-specific frameworks we considered earlier, ethics underpins the set of competencies informing each area of practice. The framework defines this as follows: 'ethical values and principles for health promotion include a belief in equity and social justice, respect for the autonomy and choice of both individuals and groups, and collaborative and consultative ways of working' (Dempsey et al., 2011, p. 8). The finer detail is presented in Box 7.1. For the full version of this framework and further details, see www.ukphr.org

---

Box 7.1 IUPHE's core competencies and professional standards for health promotion

According to this framework for practice ethical health promotion is based on a commitment to:

- Health as a human right, which is central to development;
- Respect for the rights, dignity, confidentiality and worth of individuals and groups;
- Respect for all aspects of diversity including gender, sexual orientation, age, religion, disability, ethnicity, race and cultural beliefs;
- Addressing health inequities, social justice, and prioritising the needs of those experiencing poverty and social marginalisation;
- Addressing the political, economic, social, cultural, environment, behavioural and biological determinants of health and wellbeing;
- Ensuring that health promotion action is, and what it can and cannot achieve;
- Seeking the best available information and evidence needed to implement effective policies and programmes that influence health;
- Collaboration and partnership as the basis for health promotion action;
- The empowerment of individuals and groups to build autonomy and self-respect as the basis for health promotion action;
- Sustainable development and sustainable health promotion action;
- Being accountable for the quality of one's own practice and taking responsibility for maintaining and improving knowledge and skills.

Whilst many countries were involved in the development of this international framework it was European countries played the biggest role since this region was where the work was first focussed upon. It subsequently broadened to international reach and the initial discussions about core competencies were at an international consensus meeting where global leaders in the field were involved (Barry et al., 2009). A review of the international literature on health promotion competency frameworks in 2009 found very few references 'in English language publications to health promotion and health education competencies in Africa, Asia and Latin America' concluded that 'greater effort will need to be made to include perspectives from across the globe' (Battel-Kirk et al., 2009, p. 15). It is also acknowledged that global cultural diversity, and differing values and contexts mean that developing and international code of ethics is a significant challenge, and that, as pointed out previously, most of the work that has been done on this has been dominated by the global north (Bull et al., 2012). Despite a call by Bull et al. (2012) for an international code of ethics for health promotion one has yet to emerge.

Finally, Cross et al. (2017) challenge the idea of competency frameworks on a number of grounds including their grounding in positivist, deterministic means which does not always fit with a health promotion perspective and could also therefore be called into question from an ethical point of view. Nevertheless, they note that competency frameworks for health promotion should forefront three things – the focus on health inequalities, bottom-up rather than top-down approaches, and true engagement with communities. As Bull et al. (2012) argue, 'health promotion is an ethically challenging field involving constant reflection of values across multiple cultures of what is regarded as good and bad health promotion practice' (p. 8). With this in mind it is reasonable to conclude that the possibility of reaching a true global consensus on competency frameworks is remote for now.

Sustainability

The cornerstone of health promotion, the Ottawa Charter (WHO, 1986) emphasised the need for sustainable resources and a stable eco-system as prerequisites for health alongside two key themes of this book - social justice and equity. The other fundamental conditions and resources for health cited by the charter are peace, shelter, education, food and income although the various impacts of climate change disrupt these prerequisites. Sustainability is embedded in all of the frameworks and codes of conduct that we have considered this far to some degree or another – see Box 7.2 for details.

Box 7.2   Sustainability in competency frameworks for health promotion

SHEPS (2009) – 'a commitment to sustainable development, including the adoption of a socio-ecological model of health that respects the limits of the earth's natural resources (such as land, water and sources of energy)' (p. 6).

PHSKF (2016) talks about embedding 'sustainable solutions' and ethical futures in technology for health promotion in relation to sustainability and planetary health (p. 8).

The Pan-Canadian Health Promoter Competencies and Glossary (Health Promotion Canada, 2015) – one of the underlying principles is stated as 'a dedication to sustainable development' (p. 5) and it specifies sustainable health promotion action in the development, planning, implementation and evaluation of health promotion activities.

The Australian Health Promotion Association specifically references the impacts of climate change and the implications for ecologically sustainable development under the competency that is concerned with 'mapping and analysing the environmental determinants that contribute to disease in a given community or population' (p. 13).

Sustainability is referenced in the Health Promotion New Zealand competency set twice; once with reference to the sustainability of health promotion action, and once with reference to the sustainability of coalitions and networks for health promotion action but not with specific reference to planetary health.

The IUPHE competency framework specifically mentions sustainable development and sustainable health promotion action (see Box 7.2).

As can be seen from Box 7.2 'sustainability' is talked about in two ways in the competency frameworks we have looked at. First, in relation to the sustainability of health promotion action and second, in relation to sustainable development. We now consider each in turn.

The sustainability of health promotion action

The issue of the sustainability of health promotion action is a crucial ethical one. Baldwin (2020, p. 248) asserts that sustainability in health promotion is about 'equitably and consistently enabling the promotion of health in our communities to optimum levels'. Sustainable health promotion action is ethical health promotion and has many benefits such as relative cost-effectiveness, providing evaluation opportunities to determine what works to promote health, investing in communities, and reducing long-term risks to health. However, many health promotion interventions can be criticised on the grounds of being short-lived and unsustainable for several different reasons to do with, for example, lack of political will, lack of funding and lack of engagement or simply not being fit for purpose. Nevertheless, as Bodkin and Hakimi (2020) argue, the sustainability of health promotion action is crucial to preserve intended health gains, retain community capacity, and to make the best use of resources, assets and investment. Despite this there is lack of an agreed definition of sustainability in the literature (Carstensen et al., 2018; Bodkin and Hakimi, 2020).

The sustainability of health promotion action is enhanced (or restricted) by several things. The use of integrated participatory approaches is important. In the context of tackling multiple health problems linked to the environment through an action research approach in South-Central Mexico Alamo-Hernández et al. (2019) discuss how the participation of community members, local authorities and researchers was highly beneficial resulting in 'culturally contextualised and environmentally friendly solutions' (p. 327). Collaboration has also been identified as central to the sustainability of health promotion programmes and is linked to participation and partnership (Schroeder et al., 2021). The political context is also key. As Mendes et al. (2014) point out, the political context within which health promotion programmes exist/operate may render them vulnerable to the whims of ruling parties depending on the political persuasions of those in power. In an ideal world, effective interventions would continue regardless of this which is, of course, often the most desirable and ethical outcome; however, in reality a lot of provision is subject to change depending on the politics of the time. Mendes et al. (2014, p. 72) note how micro- and macro-level policy might enhance or limit opportunities for sustainable health promotion action highlighting how the 'power context (policy environment and the power bases of stakeholders)' is an important consideration. From Denmark, Carstensen et al. (2018) consider interventions designed to promote physical health promotion in community mental health services. They identified several factors which enhance the sustainability of health promotion interventions within this context most notably that 'strong coherence and engagement of staff and management, [and having] anchor points inside and outside host organisations such as formal roles, policies and planning tools' were key (p. 503). Dattalo et al. (2017) point to the importance of organisational stability and building external partnerships for sustainability in the context of health promotion programmes designed to support older adults living in rural United States. Case Study 7.1 provides details of a paper exploring the potential

---

Case Study 7.1 Health promotion and food insecurity: exploring environmental sustainability principles to guide practice within Australia

Issue addressed: The Australian health promotion sector has made significant advances in food security over the years through recognition of social and economic factors. The incorporation of ecological determinants within health promotion practice to address food insecurity over the years through recognition of social and economic factors. The incorporation of ecological determinants within health promotion practice to address food insecurity, however, is uncommon. This paper explores the potential of health promotion to use environmental sustainability principles to guide the development of health promotion food security programs in Australia.

Methods: A mixed-methods approach guided by a pragmatic framework was adopted for this study. A national online survey ($n = 61$) and semi-structured interviews ($n = 16$) targeting Australian health promotion practitioners was utilised. Triangulation involved seven stages to develop points of convergence and corroboration of data.

Results: Practitioners were adopting principles of environmental sustainability such as integrity and biodiversity protection to guide food security practice. The use of such principles demonstrates their compatibility within health promotion practice. This study, however, reveals that environmental sustainability principles were a relatively new area of practice for health promotion practitioners.

Conclusion: The possibilities for integrating health promotion and environmental sustainability principles are promising for addressing multifaceted issues inherent within food security practice. At present, a lack of principles exists for guiding the sector to address food security that is cognisant of both human health and the environment.

So what? This study indicates a lack of integration between environmental sustainability and health promotion principles to guide food security practice. It would be pertinent for the sector to consider the development of a set of principles that considers both health promotion and environmental sustainability to ensure future food security and planetary health. Capacity building of current practitioners and preservice graduates around the use of such principles to guide practice could assist the sector in this process.

Source: Nuttman et al. (2020).

of health promotion to use environmental sustainability principles to guide the development of health promotion food security programmes in Australia.

Bodkin and Hakimi (2020) carried out a systematic review to determine the factors that inhibit and promote the sustainability of health promotion programmes. They concluded that there are several factors which influence the sustainability of health promotion action and propose that those working in health promotion should take these factors into account in the planning, developing and implementation of health promotion practice. See Box 7.3 for details. In addition, they suggest that, at the outset, there is clear identification of the components of the work that should be sustained, that sustainability should be defined 'as it relates to the context of [the programme]', and that a sustainability framework should be used to guide any intervention (Bodkin and Hakimi, 2020, p. 964). The sustainability of health promotion actions is an ethical concern which is highlighted by the problems that programme failure can bring. For example, without the active participation of communities, strategies such as community development for health promotion will be unsustainable (Warwick-Booth and Foster, 2021).

Sustainability and planetary health

As discussed earlier, sustainable development has been a key feature of the World Health Organization (WHO)'s health promotion agenda since the Ottawa Charter (WHO, 1986) and it has never been more important than it is right now. Baldwin (2020) contends that the concepts of sustainability for health promotion action are the same as for the support of people's health and planetary health – 'the interchangeability relates to the ongoing commitment, provision of policies, programs and support to make health a priority and to enable the prevention of disease and the promotion of (human and planetary health), both as a

---

Box 7.3   Factors for sustainability in health promotion action

Organisational capacity
Partnerships
Strategic planning
Funding
Fit/alignment
Programme evaluation
Capacity building
Champion
Communications
Programme implementation
Political support
Programme adaptation
Public health impacts
Socio-economic/political factors
Programme access factors
Funder priorities
Policy
Affordance
Tailored activity plans for individual clients

Source: Bodkin and Hakimi (2020)

---

human right and an "easy" and equitable option for all' (p. 251). As argued by Patrick et al. (2021), 'health promotion has a mandate to act on the ecological determinants of health' (p. 57). The two most recent international WHO health promotion conferences have highlighted sustainable development as key to health. The Shanghai Declaration (WHO, 2016), which resulted from the ninth international conference on health promotion in Shanghai, China focussed on promoting health in the 2030 Agenda for Sustainable Development and reinforced the importance of structural factors and the wider determinants of health within this context. Whilst health is only explicitly mentioned in one of the 17 Sustainable Development Goals (SDG 3: Ensure healthy lives and promote wellbeing for all at all ages) it underpins, and is necessary for, the achievement of all the other goals as well. The title of the tenth international WHO conference on health promotion was 'Health Promotion: Well-being, Equity and Sustainable Development'. This most recent conference marked the start of what was seen as a global movement on the

---

Box 7.4   The Geneva Charter for Wellbeing

The charter outlined five action areas:

1 Design an equitable economy that serves human development within planetary boundaries;
2 Create public policy for the common good;
3 Achieve universal health coverage;
4 Address the digital transformation to counteract harm and disempowerment and to strengthen the benefits; and
5 Value and preserve the planet.

Source: WHO (2021)

---

concept of wellbeing in societies and the conference re-emphasised the need for different sectors to work together without destroying the planet (WHO, 2021). See Box 7.4 for further information.

As can be seen from Box 7.3 planetary sustainability is fore fronted in the most recent international health promotion charter and, whilst it has been a concern for some time now, health promotion interventions have arguably only more recently started to take into account impact of environmental concerns such as climate change on human health experience (Patrick and Kingsley, 2019) despite a recognition of the significance of the natural environment for human health for several decades now (Patrick et al., 2021). It is well evidenced that the impact of climate change and environmental degradation is experienced more significantly by the most disadvantaged and less well-off in our world. The most affected are in the least-powerful positions to effect change. This results in worsening health inequities which is an ethical challenge and calls into question the issue of social justice also. Climate change is a 'wicked'[1] problem which means that 'the interwoven social, political, and cultural differences across countries make the issue of climate change difficult to address on a global scale' (Sun and Yang, 2016, npn). Despite the complexity of adopting such approaches writers such as Patrick and Kingsley (2019) advocate for the adoption of holistic ecological models to guide health promotion practice. Wicked issues such as climate change and the destruction of the natural environment can feel far removed from the day-to-day reality of people's lives, especially for those who are struggling the most, such that individual action can be rendered relatively meaningless. Health promoters therefore have a duty to work to create change not just at the individual level but, more importantly, at local and structural

Box 7.5 Strategies for health promotion practitioners

Downstream approaches include:

- Encouraging the use of public transport (buses, trains, trams) and active transport (cycling, walking);
- Encouraging participation in active projects such as community gardening;
- Encouraging participations in sustainable food practices and consumption;
- Encouraging contact with nature and interaction with(in) green and blue spaces promoting nature as a key setting for health promotion;
- Embed environmental issues in health promotion programme planning;
- Develop interventions that directly address climate change.

Upstream approaches include:

- Advocating for mitigation and adaptation at national and international levels;
- Focusing on environmental and ecological issues as well as equity;
- Influencing and creating healthy public policy such as sustainable transport.

Source: Patrick and Kingsley (2019, 2021)

levels. Box 7.5 provides some details about what health promoters can do to tackle climate change using downstream and upstream approaches.

Lutz et al. (2020) point out the importance of raising awareness of the threat of climate change to human health in the education of health practitioners arguing also that they need to be trained in sustainable development. Ideally the subject of sustainable development should be embedded within the curriculum for everyone who studies health promotion and associated subject areas. Lutz et al. (2020) contend that the subjects of social determinants of health, inter-sectorial action and multilevel governance are examples of where the relationships between health promotion and sustainability can be explored and appreciated. They conclude that 'training health professionals to sustainable development represents a major strategy to respond to climate change and its health impacts' (npn).

Ecological approaches to health promotion

Ecological approaches to promoting health take into account the interactions between people and their environment. As Richard and Gauvin (2017, p. 85) point out, 'contrary to traditional ecology, which highlight[s] the physical features of environment, the ecological approach used in health promotion is more socio-ecological in nature and focuses more centrally on the social, organizational, and cultural components of the environment'. They go on to argue that the integration ecological principles in health promotion practice is possible. We would go further and say it is not just possible but necessary. As Smith and Nersesian (2023, pntbc) argue, 'because local environments are inextricably linked to the earth's ecosystems, health promotion exists within the context of a healthy planet. Recognising and acknowledging that people's actions affect the planet, and the health of the planet affects people's health is essential to achieving health and wellbeing outcomes'. Patrick et al. (2021 p. 475) therefore advocate for 'paradigmatic shifts in health promotion thinking and acting in the context of climate change'.

Returning to ethical considerations it is notable, as Patrick et al. (2011) argues, that the core values of health promotion 'can translate into action in the area of climate change and environmental sustainability' (p. 476). In addition to the three key values that form the main themes of this book – equity, social justice and empowerment – these also include a socio-ecological model of health, respect for cultural diversity, a commitment to sustainable development, and community participation in the health promotion planning process as outlined by Allegrante et al. (2009). The unequal impact of climate change has been acknowledged; however, there are other features of modernity that cause a lack of equity. For example, whilst technological advances increase individual opportunity and agency to shape private worlds, these tend to be unevenly distributed/available and those who have access to such means are therefore able to exercise a level of power over their own lives (and others) that the less fortunate cannot (Cross et al., 2017). Examples such as these highlight ethical concerns to do with equity, social justice and empowerment. They also emphasise the collective responsibility that is required to address such issues.

Redistributive policy

The final issue under discussion in this chapter is redistributive policy. The United Nations Economic and Social Commission for Western Asia (ESCWA, 2020) note that redistributive policies are 'an essential component of strategies for reducing inequality and promoting sustainable development in its three dimensions: economic, social and environmental' (npn). Redistributive policy is not just about the more equitable allocation of wealth, it is also about other forms of capital such as land and income-generating capacity for greater equality. One example of redistributive policy is Universal Basic Income. Please see Case Study 7.2 for further details. Much has been written about various forms of redistributive policy all of which bring to the fore different values and perspectives. There is not the capacity here to outline all the different scenarios and debates so we will focus on proportionate universalism. Work by Sir Michael Marmot and his team over the past two decades has shown a stark social gradient in health (e.g. Marmot, 2010 and Marmot et al., 2020). The social gradient of health is that the lower down the social strata a person is, the more likely they are to experience adverse health outcomes. The most deprived and disadvantaged fair the worst (Francis-Oliviero et al., 2020). As a result, Marmot (2010) is a strong advocate of proportionate universalism whereby actions to tackle

---

Case Study 7.2   Universal Basic Income

Universal Basic Income (UBI) is a state scheme where every adult in a said population is given a set amount of money regularly regardless of whether they work or not, or are *able* to work or not. It is an unconditional payment not linked to any other income or wealth. Those who advocate for UBI argue that it could reduce poverty, as well as improving health, wellbeing and income security. Sometimes referred to as Citizen's Basic Income, proposals of UBI spark fierce debate about the advantages and challenges of such a measure. From a health and wellbeing perspective it is argued that the introduction of UBI would remove (or at least reduce) the stress of repeated means-testing and also address the potential stigma and discrimination that those receiving state benefits might experience. In addition, others have emphasised the 'emancipatory nature' of having a basic income in that it 'gives people the possibility to be creative, is empowering and diminishes financial insecurity' (Kangas et al., 2019). Finland has carried out a basic income experiment which took place for two years during 2017–2018. Preliminary findings suggested that those receiving the basic income reported higher levels of general wellbeing and experienced fewer problems related to health and stress. These findings were further supported in a survey that took place at the end of the experiment – there was 'a statistically significant difference in favour of basic-income recipients [...] in their subjective perceptions of health and stress, and their trust in other people and institutions' (Van Parijs, 2020, p. 3).

Reflection on Practice 7.2

Reflecting on the discussion and debates this book has presented, and your own personal values and principles, what would an ethical future in health promotion look like to you? Consider the issues of equity, empowerment and social justice which have been key themes throughout this book. What things would need to change at the micro, marco and meso levels in order to promote a more ethical future for everyone in terms of health experience and health outcomes? You could also consider these questions in relation to the issue of planetary health.

---

the social gradient in health are universal (for everyone) but 'with a scale and intensity that is proportionate to the level of disadvantage' (Macdonald et al., 2014, p. 1). Proportionate universalism is about improving the health of the worst off in our communities as well as reducing the social gradient by improving health for everyone. The basic idea is that those in greater need receive greater attention and resources the purpose being to reduce health inequalities. Zhang et al. (2022) note that proportionate universalism is a promising strategy for promoting health equity. The principles of proportionate universalism can be seen in redistributive policies such as progressive taxation. One of the advantages of proportionate universalism, from an ethical point of view, is that it does not target specific groups or people (an approach strongly advocated by Marmot, 2015) so helping to avoid stigmatisation. As a final task please take some time to carry out Reflection on Practice 7.2. This will give an opportunity to reflect on some of the key issues that this book has presented in relation to health promotion ethics.

Summary

SHEPS Cymru and Shaping the Future (2009) made the important point some years ago that the promotion of health requires innovation and, whilst we need to take the underpinning values and principles into account, they should not 'unnecessarily' restrict innovative ways of working. In this chapter we have considered what an ethical future for health promotion might look like. Specifically, we have focussed on issues of sustainability – both in terms of the sustainability of health promotion actions and in terms of planetary health. No doubt, an ethical future for health promotion will require that those working in health promotion find innovative and creative solutions for promoting people's health in a likely increasingly complex and challenging world. Those solutions will need to take into account the health of our planet as inextricably linked with our own.

Key points

- An ethical foundation is critical to inform and underpin the values of health promotion practice and this is reflected different frameworks for health promotion.
- Sustainability is a key ethical issue in health promotion, in terms of the sustainability of health promotion interventions and, for example, the judicious use of resources and assets. Redistributive policies are one example of strategy to tackle health inequity.
- Health promotion has an important part to play in planetary health as the health of people and the planet are inextricably linked.

Further reading

Kohler, P. (2015) *Redistributive Policies for Sustainable Development: Looking at the Role of Assets and Equity.* DESA Working Paper No. 139. ST/ESA/2015/DWP/139. Retrieved from un.org/esa/desa/papers/2015/wp139_2015.pdf
This substantial paper explores the relationships between redistribution, equity and sustainable development with an emphasis on social and environmental dimensions. It sets out several different avenues for redistributive polices to promote greater equity, economic power and sustainable development.

Note

1 '"Wicked" is the term used to describe some of the most challenging and complex issues of our time, many of which threaten human health' (Walls, 2018, p. 1). Arguably climate change is the wickedest problem of all.

References

Alamo-Hernández, U., Espinosa-García, A.C., Rangel-Flores, H., Farías, P., Hernández-Bonilla, D., Cortez-Lugo, M. et al. (2019) Environmental health promotion of a contaminated site in Mexico. *EcoHealth*, 16, 317–329.
Allegrante, J.P., Barry, M.M., Airhihenbuwa, O., Auld, M.E., Battel-Kirk, B., Collins, L. et al. (2009) *Toward Domains of Core Competency for Building Global Capacity in Health Promotion: The Galway Consensus Conference Statement.* Galway Conference, Draft April 2009.
Baldwin, L. (2020) Chapter 12: Sustaining the practice of health promotion. In Fleming, M. and Baldwin, L. (Eds.), *Health Promotion in the 21st Century: New Approaches to Achieving Health for All.* London, Allen & Unwin.
Barry, M., Allegante, J.P., Lamarre, M., Auld, M. and Taub, A. (2009) The Galway Consensus Conference: International collaboration on the development of core competencies for health promotion and health education. *Global Health Promotion*, 16 (2), 5–11.
Battel-Kirk, B., Barry, M., Taub, A. and Lysoby, L. (2009) A review of the international literature on health promotion competencies: Identifying frameworks and core competencies. *Global Health Promotion*, 16 (2), 12–20.

Bodkin, A. and Hakimi, S. (2020) Sustainable by design: A systematic review of factors for health promotion program sustainability. *BMC Public Health*, 20, 964. https://doi.org/10.1186/s12889-020-09091-9

Bull, T., Riggs, E. and Nchogu, S.N. (2012) Does health promotion need a Code of Ethics? Results from an IUHPE mixed method study. *Global Health Promotion*, 19 (3), 8–20.

Carstensen, K., Kousgaard, M. and Burau, V. (2018) Sustaining an intervention for physical health promotion in community mental health services: A multi-site case study. *Health and Social Care in the Community*, 27, 502–515.

Cross, R., Davis, S. and O'Neil, I. (2017) *Health Promotion: Theoretical and Critical Perspectives*. Cambridge, Polity.

Dattalo, M., Wise, M., Ford, J., Abramson, H. and Mahoney, B. (2017) Essential resources for implementation and sustainability of evidence-based health promotion programs: A mixed methods multi-site case study. *Journal of Community Health*, 42, 358–368.

Dempsey, C., Battel-Kirk, B. and Barry, M. (2011) *The CompHP CORE COMPETENCIES FRAMEWORK FOR HEALTH PROMOTION HANDBOOK*. Ireland, EAHC.

ESCWA (2020) *Redistributive Policies*. [Internet] Retrieved from archive. unescwa.org

Francis-Oliviero, F., Cambon, L., Wittwer, J., Marmot, M. and Alla, F. (2020) Theoretical and practical challenges of proportionate universalism: A review. *Revista Panamericana de Salud Publica*, 44, e110. https://doi.org/10.26633/RPSP.2020.110

Health Promotion Canada (2015) The Pan-Canadian health promoter competencies and glossary. Retrieved from www.healthpromotioncanada.ca

Health Promotion Forum of New Zealand (2012) *Health Promotion Competencies for Aotearoa*. Auckland, Health Promotion Form of New Zealand.

IUHPE (2016) *Core competencies and professional standard for health promotion*. International Union of Health Promotion and Education. Retrieved from www.ukphr.org

Kangas, O., Jauhiainen, S., Simanainen, M. and Ylikännö (Eds.) (2019) *The Basic Income Experiment 2017–2018 in Finland. Preliminary Results*. Helsinki, Ministry of Social Affairs and Health.

Lutz, A., Pasche, M. and Zűrcher, K. (2020) Integrating sustainability in professionals' training in the field of health promotion and prevention. *16th World Congress on Public Health 2020*, Rome, 12th–16th October.

Macdonald, W., Beeston, C. and McCullough, S. (2014) *Proportionate Universalism and Health Inequalities*. Edinburgh, NHS Health Scotland.

Marmot, M. (2010) *Fair Society, Healthy Lives: Strategic Review of Health Inequalities in England Post-2010*. London, Institute of Health Equity.

Marmot, M. (2015) Commentary: Mental health and public health. *International Journal of Epidemiology*, 43, 293–296.

Marmot, M., Allen, J., Boyce, T., Goldblatt, P. and Morrison, J. (2020) *Health Equity in England: The Marmot Review 10 Years on*. London, Institute of Health Equity.

Mendes, R., Plaza, V. and Wallerstein, N. (2014) Sustainability and power in health promotion: Community-based participatory research in a reproductive health policy case study in New Mexico. *Global Health Promotion*, 23 (1), 61–74.

Nuttman, S., Patrick, R., Townsend, M. and Lawson, J. (2020) Health promotion and food insecurity: Exploring environmental sustainability principles to guide practice within Australia. *Health Promotion Journal of Australia*, 31, 6.

Patrick, R., Capetola, T., Townsend, M. and Nuttman, S. (2011) Health promotion and climate change: Exploring the core competencies required for action. *Health Promotion International*, 27 (4). https://doi.org/10.1093/heapro/dar055

Patrick, R., Henderson-Wilson, C. and Ebden, M. (2021) Exploring the co-benefits of environmental volunteering for human and planetary health promotion. *Health Promotion Journal of Australia*, 33, 57–67.

Patrick, R. and Kingsley, J. (2019) Health promotion and sustainability programmes in Australia: Barriers and enabler to evaluation. *Global Health Promotion*, 26 (2), 82–92.

PHSKF (2016) *Public Health Skills and Knowledge Framework*. London, Public Health England.

Richard, L. and Gauvin, L. (2017) Chapter 5: Building and implementing ecological health promotion interventions. In Rootman, I., Pederson, A., Frohlich, K.L. and Dupéré, S. (Eds.) *Health Promotion in Canada: New Perspectives on Theory, Practice, Policy and Research*, 4th Edn. Toronto, Canadian Scholars.

Schroeder, K., Deatrick, J.A., Klusaritz, H., Bowman, C., Williams, T.T., Lee, J. et al. (2021) Using a community workgroup approach to increase access to physical activity in an under-resourced urban community. *Health Promotion Practice*, 21 (1), 5–11.

SHEPS Cymru and Shaping the Future (2009) A Framework for Ethical Health Promotion: Draft. SHEPS and Shaping the Future.

Smith, L. and Nersesian, P. (2023) Chapter 13: Reimagining child and family health education and health promotion through a planetary health Lens. In: Cross, R. (Ed.), *Health Promotion and Health Education for Nurses*. London, Sage.

Somerset, S., Robinson, P. and Kelsall, H. (2016) *Foundation Competencies for Public Health Graduates in Australia*. Council of Academic Public Health Institutions, Australia.

Sun, J. and Yang, K. (2016) The wicked problem of climate change: A new approach based on social mess and fragmentation. *Sustainability*, 8 (12). https://doi.org/10.3390/su8121312

Van den Broucke, S. (2021) Strengthening health promotion practice: Capacity development for a transdisciplinary field. *Global Health Promotion*, 28 (4). https://doi.org/10.1177/1757959211061751

Van Parijs, P. (2020) Basic income: Finland's final verdict. *Social Europe*, 7th May, 2020. [Internet] Retrieved from acdc2007.free.fr/vanparijs520.pdf

Walls, H. (2018) Wicked problems and a 'wicked' solution. *Globalization and Health*, 14, 34. https://doi/org/10.1186/s12992-018-0353-x

Warwick-Booth, L. and Foster, S. (2021) Chapter 2: People, power and communities. In Cross, R., Warwick-Booth, L., Rowlands, S., Woodall, J., O'Neil, I. and Foster, S.(Eds.), *Health Promotion: Global Principles and Practice*. 2nd Ed. Wallingford, CABI.

134   *Towards an ethical future in health promotion*

Woodall, J. and Cross, R. (2022) *Essentials of Health Promotion*. London, Sage.
World Health Organization (WHO) (1986) *The Ottawa Charter*. Geneva, World Health Organization.
World Health Organization (WHO) (2016) *The Shanghai Declaration*. Geneva, World Health Organization.
World Health Organization (WHO) (2021) *The Geneva Charter for Well-being*. Geneva, World Health Organization.
Zhang, J.H., Ramke, J., Jan, C., Bascaran, C., Mwangi, N. and Furtado, J.M. et al. (2022) Advancing the Sustainable Development Goals through improving eye health: A scoping review. *Lancet Planet Health*, 6, e270–280.

Index

Note: *Italicized* and **bold** pages refer to figures and tables respectively.

Printed and bound by CPI Group (UK) Ltd, Croydon, CR0 4YY

17/10/2024

01775670-0001